The Ultimate Guide to Hemp CBD Oil

Complete Guide to Dealing with Anxiety, Depression, Diseases, Pain Relief and CBD Legality Improve Health and Happiness Using this Miraculous Oil

Jake Wood

Additionally, the information found on the following pages is intended for informational purposes only and should thus be considered, universal. As befitting its nature, the information presented is without assurance regarding its continued validity or interim quality. Trademarks that is mentioned are done without written consent and can in no way be considered an endorsement from the trademark holder.

Table of Contents

Introduction

Congratulations on getting *The Ultimate Guide to Hemp CBD Oil: Complete Guide to Dealing with Anxiety, Depression, Diseases, Pain Relief and CBD Legality - Improve Health and Happiness Using This Miraculous Oil* and thank you for doing so.

People around the world have been awakened by the sound of this wonder oil and it is high time we also get on board. Getting this book places profound knowledge on the wonders of the CBD Oil in your hands. This wisdom will help you and your loved ones manage pain, disease symptoms, and other conditions with ease.

Majority of the people around the world are choosing to tow the health path by avoiding synthetic products, highly processed foods, and excessive sugars in a bid to protect their health. Many of them are trying to trace back their steps by going back to the basics of life, to what life was before the onset of gadgets, technology, and other changes that disrupted life. Many are now exercising and avoiding exposure to harmful items, but sadly, some still depend on modern synthetic solutions to health problems while natural solutions exist.

To that end, the following chapters will discuss CBD oil as the natural solution to the majority of the health problems the world has today. You will understand how CBD oil is made, the plants from which it is sourced, and different methods used to extract it. You will also learn how to ingest it, where to buy it, how to buy it, and what to look out for as side effects. This book will delve into details discussing the use of CBD oil in treating and repressing the symptoms of many chronic diseases and conditions, with an accompanying chapter of testimonials on the successes of CBD oil. This book is sure to leave you astounded at the wonders of this oil.

There are plenty of books on this subject on the market, so thanks again for choosing this one! Every effort was made to ensure it is full of as much useful information as possible. Please enjoy!

Chapter 1: CBD Oil

Cannabidiol (CBD) oil is becoming quite popular in the United States, even in states where the use of marijuana is illegal. Part of the reason for this increased awareness is the push and pulls between promoters and those who are against the use of CBD oil. Supporters claim that the oil has a number of health benefits, while the opposition is quick to issue a caution on the health threats that CBD oil could bring.

Claims that CBD potentially has benefits that could benefit every individual user are also rousing much interest because what was previously only recommended for critically ill patients is now universally used. In addition, the oil is increasingly available and consumers have the opportunity to test it for themselves. So, what is this mysterious oil?

CBD oil is oil that has CBD infused. CBD, in itself, is a chemical compound in the cannabis plant. It is one of the groups of 104 compounds called the cannabinoids. CBD occurs naturally in the cannabis plant and when extracted, is mixed with a carrier oil from either coconuts or the hemp seed. This mixture makes the CBD oil. A number of compounds including the most popular cannabinoid, tetrahydrocannabinol (THC), are psychoactive, but CBD is not. You would not get 'high' by consuming it.

Just like other products that are extracted from something primary, the composition of cannabis oils relies on the process of making the extract and the elements that are in the plant itself. Some extraction processes may produce oil with some level of THC having not been able to separate the two because the production of CBD oil is not regulated. However, properly sourced and processed CBD oil should not be psychoactive.

If both CBD and THC come from cannabis sativa, what makes them different? The difference is that CBD is processed from the hemp. Hemp is a form of the cannabis plant with a high CBD concentration and manufacturers prefer sourcing CBD from it to increase the chances of producing high-quality oil.

There is a distinct difference between marijuana and hemp despite coming from the same plant, the cannabis sativa. The difference is that farmers planting marijuana have been growing their plants selectively over the years, in a bid to ensure that they contained the highest THC levels and other compounds. These compounds are said to produce a specific smell or to have an intended effect on the flowers of the plant. However, farmers growing the hemp version have not made any significant modifications. Therefore, extracting fluid from the hemp plant is sure to produce a lot of CBD than THC.

The hemp plant is also excitingly earth-friendly because unlike many commercial crops, the plant does not require any pesticides, being naturally resistant. In addition, rather than depleting all the resources in the soil, hemp revitalizes it.

CBD Oil and Hemp Oil Are Different

The fact that CBD oil and Hemp oil are produced from the same hemp does not make them alike. Hemp oil is derived from hemp seeds and does not contain much of the cannabidiol compounds. In contrast, CBD oil is extracted from the entire hemp plant, not just the seeds. There are also thousands of hemp varieties, but the kinds used to produce CBD oil will often have high cannabidiol concentrations.

Hemp oil and CBD oil are also different based on their extraction processes. Hemp oil is cold pressed from hemp or cannabis seeds, which contain 30% oil. In cold pressing, the seeds are de-shelled and once the seed is off, the seeds are chilled and squeezed for the oil to be extracted. Despite its source, cannabis or hemp, the oil does not contain any psychoactive compounds.

Although CBD oil can be extracted from both the cannabis and hemp plants, the laws in many regions limit the amount of THC that can be found in CBD oil, making it easier and cheaper to extract it from the CBD-rich hemp. As a result, CBD production primarily leans on the hemp. In addition, manufacturers use cutting-edge supercritical carbon dioxide in the extraction process.

Therefore, the parent material and the extraction processes differentiate between CBD oil and hemp oil. The parts used during the extraction process also make a significant difference.

How CBD Oil Works

CBD oil works in a number of ways as described below:

First, CBD acts as an allosteric regulator for a number of receptor sites in the body. Allosteric regulation is the process of balancing or modulating an enzyme by binding an effector molecule at a different site rather than at the enzyme's active site. A regulator does this by modifying the shape of certain receptors, altering their ability to respond to neurotransmitters.

The human body already engages in the production of some cannabinoids naturally, making available CB1 and CB2 receptors. CB1 receptors are located in the brain while CB2 are mostly found in the body's immune system. CB1 receptors control functions such as emotions, pain, body movement and coordination, memories, thinking, and appetite, among other functions whose control is the brain. THCs typically attach to CB1 receptors. CB2 receptors, on the other hand, affect pain and inflammation. For a while, researchers believed that CBD attaches to CB2 receptors, but recent studies have been proving otherwise, indicating that CBD does not need either of the receptors. Instead, it points the body towards using its own cannabinoids.

CBD fights GPR55 receptors. The GPR55 receptors are dispersed in the brain, the cerebellum in particular, and they work to regulate blood pressure and bone density. However, once these receptors are activated, they promote the growth of cancer cells. For this reason, it is important to supplement

CBDD for persons with high blood pressure, cancer, and osteoporosis.

CBD positively modulates delta and mu opioid receptors, which means that it heightens the receptors' ability to receive endogenous enkephalins that work to reduce the intensity of pain naturally, and thereby, improve the quality of life. In reverse, CBD is also a negative modulator to the CB1 receptor as mentioned, because it reduces the receptor's ability to bind with THC. This is the reason cultivars with a high CBD level are used to alleviate THC side effects.

When taken in high dosages, CBD stimulates the 5-ht1A receptor. This receptor regulates addiction, sleep, nausea, appetite, anxiety, and vomiting. The raw form of CBD, called CBDA, particularly indicates a higher affinity for the 5-ht1A receptor than CBD does.

CBD also triggers PPAR-gamma receptors. These receptors are located in the nucleus of cells and are involved in the regulation of functions like dopamine release, lipid uptake, the breakdown of amyloid plaque, and insulin sensitivity. This is the reason why taking CBD is considered important for people with Alzheimer's disease, diabetes, and schizophrenia.

Lastly, CBD also stimulates TRPV1 receptors. These receptors are involved in the regulation of temperature, pain, and inflammation in the body. TRPV1 receptors are particularly targeted by capsaicin, anandamide, and various cannabinoid compounds like CBDV, THC, CBC, CBN, and CBG.

Evidence to Prove How CBD Works

Proof of how CBD oil works are best observed through an evaluation of how CBD interacts with different receptors in the body to lessen disease symptoms. Various scientific studies and circumstantial evidence have successfully proven that CBD oil is an important component that helps to lessen the symptoms of a number of illnesses. Although these illnesses are a broad spectrum, the common target of influence is the endogenous cannabinoid system, also called the endocannabinoid system. This endocannabinoid system, named after the parent cannabis plant, consists of molecules and receptors that reside in the glands, brain, organs, and other cells in the body. This system is responsible for various body functions including temperature control, motor coordination, brain and nerve tissue, sleep, mood, memory, metabolism, hunger, and appetite.

Products in which THC is absent are not within the U.S. Drug Enforcement Agency's (DEA) scope according to the Controlled Substances Act, which indicates that people are free to trade and consume anything without THC like CBD. This is possibly the reason CBD products are increasingly popular and more socially accepted. In 2016, Forbes projected that by 2020, the CBD industry will have grown tremendously, reaching at least $2.2 billion.

That said, cannabinoids are important structures and heavily affect the endocannabinoid system by influencing body receptors either directly or indirectly. In the event the endocannabinoid system is frail, the cannabinoid, in this case, the CBD, increase the functioning of the receptors, enabling them to work optimally. The cannabinoids link up the organs and the nervous system, balancing the mind and the body perfectly.

Chapter 2: The History of the Use of CBD Oil

Since the frenzy on the benefits of CBD oil has only been here a little while, many assume that CBD is a new innovative supplement, but CBD oil and its use go way back. In actuality, CBD has had a rich history with humans, dating back to 4000 B.C.

The early people grew cannabis plants. However, the mode of cultivation and the usage made the difference between the two most prominent cannabis strains – marijuana and hemp. Marijuana was used for recreational purposes while industrial hemp was used in the production of papers, textile, and ropes. Early Chinese records even portray the hemp plant as one of the primary crops at the time. Beginning from the time of the primitive societies during the Qin and Han dynasties, a lot of focus and attention was put into the seeding, tilling, and processing of the hemp plant and its husbandry advanced quickly. China began to recognize hemp as one of its main crops.

Cultivation of hemp continued into the 1533s, at a time when King Henry VIII required farmers to set aside a section of their farms for cultivation of hemp. Those who did not comply had to pay a hefty fine. This was also the case during colonial America when all farmers were required to grow hemp by law. In fact, Founding Father Thomas Jefferson instructed farmers to reserve an acre of their best grounds to cultivate hemp. Interestingly, the colonial masters got into the country using boats that used hemp ropes. The constitution of America was also drafted on paper made from hemp. Therefore, at the time, cannabis had grown and its use spread across the world, both recreational and industrial uses.

Although cannabis has been around a while and even aided in the development of civilization, the medicinal aspects of CBD are only now becoming a 'thing'. It is important to note that scientists began to ask questions on the possible medical value of cannabis in 1533, but they were only able to extract CBD itself in the mid-1950s. Not much research could have been done before the scientists were able to extract the CBD compound. The extraction process helped lay to rest questions on whether CBD was psychoactive since it was drawn from the cannabis plant. This investigation began the legal battles surrounding CBD, which even today are yet to be resolved fully.

As early as 1563, questions had already started coming up as people desired to know the true composition of the hemp and marijuana plants. Garcia da Orta, a Portuguese physician realized that when his servants took the cannabis plant, they did not feel like working, appeared to be very happy, and developed an astonishing appetite for food. Around that time also, Li Shizhen, a Chinese doctor, wrote about the anti-nausea effect of cannabis. A story is also told of Queen Victoria. It says that she would smoke cannabis whenever she had menstrual cramps and this would ease her pain. These seemingly insignificant notes became the basis for research into the components of cannabis and hemp plants, which has brought about the knowledge of their properties and distinctions, as we know them today.

Roger Adams, a Harvard University alumnus, was the first chemist to extract CBD from the cannabis plant in 1940. However, when he did it, he was not aware of what he had done or of the chemical compound he had extracted. It was not until many years later that he and other scientists realized the value of the groundbreaking work he had done that they set out to examine the possible CBD benefits.

The modern history of the CBD we are learning about today began in 1946 when Dr. Walter S. Loewe tried the CBD on animals in the lab. These tests provided proof that CBD did not alter the user's mental state. In that same year, Dr. Raphael Mechoulam came up with the CBD's 3D structure and got him accreditation and recognition as the scientists who discovered CBD. More research on the abilities and effects of CBD continued into the 1960s until the time when British Pharmacopoeia released the first CBD oil tinctures for therapeutic purposes.

As research progressed in the decades that followed, Dr.Mechoulam made another unprecedented breakthrough in the history of CBD in 1980. He conducted a study, which showed that CBD would be instrumental in treating epilepsy. This research was followed by a highly publicized story of Charlotte Figi, a young girl whose rare seizure disorder was treated using a CBD potent treatment.

The story was followed by a battle as the fight for the legalization of CBD ensued. In the 1950s, all 50 states outlawed CBD. However, medical and scientific research brought back questions on the legality of CBD. These questions became the foundations for some of the landmark events in the history of CBD. For example, the US government patented the first CBD-based patent on October 2, 2003, while in 2017, the FDA began taking steps towards legalization and approval of CBD for medical purposes.

Below are a summary and a chronological timeline to illustrate the CBD journey, from discovery in the 1940s to the shelves in 2018.

1940: Roger Adams extracts CBD from marijuana without knowing
Adams had spent years researching marijuana and when he succeeded in isolating CBD from the plant, he did not describe its chemical structure and credit was given to Raphael Mechoulam who did.

1946: Dr. Loewe conducts his preliminary CBD test on animals in his lab
Dr. Loewe ran tests on mice and rabbits using cannabinoids CBD, CBN, and THC. He found that THC caused the mice to be in some sort of a trance, while CBD did not affect behavior in any observable way, which showed that CBD lacks

psychotropic abilities.

1964: Raphael Mechoulam describes CBD's chemical structure
This Israeli scientist determined the chemical structure of CBD in his lab at the Hebrew University of Jerusalem in 1963

The late 1960s: Mechoulam starts testing different cannabinoids on primates
These tests helped prove that THC, and not CBD, sedated and intoxicated the brain after consumption

The mid-1970s: British Pharmacopoeia releases the first CBD tincture
The potential medical uses of CBD became known after Mechoulam released his findings on the active elements in CBD. British Pharmacopoeia released the first cannabis tincture containing full spectrum CBD oil for therapeutic purposes.

1978: New Mexico acknowledges the medical potentials of cannabis
New Mexico was the first state to approve the use of cannabis products for medicinal purposes.

1980: Mechoulam joins researchers from South America in a study to determine the relationship between CBD and epilepsy
Mechoulam worked with researchers from Sao Paulo Medicine Faculty of Santa Casa in Brazil to conduct a study of 16 subjects with epilepsy, to determine how they would feel after receiving CBD. The subjects felt better and did not have any side effects. This experiment became a major breakthrough in the study of medical benefits of marijuana.

The 1980s: Mechoulam's research on the efficiency of CBD on epilepsy received no recognition
Not even one of the medical or pharmaceutical industries in America took notice of the findings of the study. This study should have sparked support from across the world.

1996: California legalizes medical marijuana

California was the first US state to legalize medical use and this decision paved the way for other states, which quickly followed. By the end of the century in the year 2000, Alaska, Oregon, Maine, Washington, Nevada, Colorado, and Hawaii had made the move too.

2003: The US government patents the neuroprotective characteristics of CBD

This move by the government meant that it recognized CBD's medicinal qualities although it still did not remove CBD oil from the scheduled narcotics list

2013: Charlotte Figi's story goes viral

People learned that Figi had gotten relief when the hundreds of grand mal seizures she experienced every week were stopped after she used a cannabis plant with a high CBD concentration as the last resort.

2014: A number of states legalize CBD oil

The states of Tennessee, Wisconsin, North Carolina, Alabama, South Carolina, Missouri, Mississippi, Florida, Kentucky, Iowa, and Utah passed legislation allowing its citizens to use medical CBD oil.

2017: FDA takes initial steps towards recognizing CBD oil as medicine

Plans are underway to recognize CBD oil as a drug that physicians across the country can prescribe. It will be the first cannabis product to gain FDA approval and acknowledgment.

Chapter 3: How to Buy CBD Oil

Many people are increasingly aware of the negative effects of the majority of prescription drugs in the market and are consciously making efforts to reduce the number of prescription drugs they take. A significant proportion is now turning towards natural products to help manage conditions like anxiety, pain, and inflammation. CBD is quickly gaining popularity as the ultimate health solution and many people are purchasing it.

When buying CBD oil, you need accurate and current information about it. CBD is one of the most misjudged products in the market and there are many misguiding sources of information mixed together with accurate versions. Therefore, to have the right information, you will need to dig deep, to get reliable information. However, this book has done the job for you. It has compiled reliable information scattered across the web and in other sources to bring you a comprehensive guide to help you in your endeavor to purchase CBD oil.

Purchasing CBD Oil

CBD oil comes in different forms and identifying the right one to pick can be a challenge to first-time buyers. Many people confuse CBD oil with THC, the psychoactive cannabis ingredient. Even those in the know, who understand the difference between THC and CBD, often find that they need guidance because there still are many factors involved when purchasing CBD oil such as strength, concentrations, product type, purity, volume, brands, and of course, your need.

Here are some steps you need to follow when purchasing CBD oil

Chose Hemp-Based and not Marijuana-Based oil
When purchasing CBD oil, keep in mind that manufacturers

use either the hemp plant or the marijuana plant to make the oil. Oil made from the marijuana is illegal in the United States and its transportation across state lines is also prohibited. Therefore, to avoid involvement in illegal trade, ensure that you only select hemp-based oil products.

Decide on the quantity you need

It is always better to determine the amount of a particular substance you will need before making a decision on how much of it to purchase to prevent buying too much of it or making repeat transactions. Many consumers prefer going by the recommended dosage when purchasing drugs. However, when it comes to determining the amount of CBD to consume, popularly called a serving, the FDA has placed restrictions and guidelines to manufacturers indicating that they are to refrain from recommending CBD servings. The FDA placed this directive because it requires that CBD oil is treated only as a food product and not as a medical product, and if sellers make recommendations, they would be implying that CBD is a treatment for health conditions, while CBD is not an approved cure or treatment.

Therefore, when purchasing CBD oil, you will need to calculate your own requirements. For example, if you need to use 30mg CBD per serving, taking it twice per day, you will need to make provisions to support you taking 60mg CBD per day. Therefore, if you buy a bottle containing 300mg CBD, know that you will be buying 5 days' worth of oil. For many people, five days consumption is not adequate to reap the full benefits of the oil. You may want to purchase oil to last at least a month.

The Intake Method

CBD oil products will come in the form of capsules, drops, gummies, and others. All these product forms carry the same hemp extract. It will not matter the form in which you get your product. Therefore, the decision on which form of CBD oil to choose will solely rely on your preference.

Having established that the intended product is hemp-based,

determined the amount you need and the preferred intake method, it is now time to choose from among a number of different CBD oils available in the market. The opinions of others through consumer reviews and the prices of the oils could distract you and prevent you from getting the right product. To prevent this from happening, you need a clear guide to help cut through the turbulent waters of opinion and market prices.

Here's how to get the right products:

1. Get to know the basics

To begin, get to know where the hemp was grown to understand what it may contain.

The hemp plant is a bio-accumulator, which means that it absorbs everything, both good and bad elements, from the water, the air, and the soil. Organically grown hemp is better because based on its composition, it can be traced back to where it was grown. It also does not contain toxic elements like heavy metals, herbicides, and pesticides. These harmful elements are linked to serious conditions and diseases like soft tissue sarcoma, leukemia, multiple myeloma, non-Hodgkin lymphoma, and a number of cancers. To avoid these dangers, only seek out hemp products made from organic plants.

The only way to be certain that the CBD oil you are buying is pure and does not contain foreign elements is to buy oil from a transparent seller, one whose source can be traced back to a farm, preferably in the United States.

2. The level of THC in the CBD oil is important

While CBD oil is non-psychoactive, it is likely to contain traces of THC depending on the extraction methods that were used. Some consumers do not mind having more than a few THC traces, but if you work with heavy machinery, can be subjected to drug tests at work, or you fall into other special categories, you want to consume none or the bare minimal THC level possible. According to the law, CBD oil is considered legal only if its THC level is less than 0.03%.

Therefore, as you select CBD oil, ensure that you select one whose THC level is zero or only contains minimal traces of THC. Kindly note that most reputable sellers will produce oil that does not contain any THC, and therefore, if you hold any reservations regarding even the smallest traces of TCH, it is best to stick to reputable oils.
The benefits of pure and clean CBD oil is that you will not fail any drug tests, there will be no mind-altering effects, and it complies with the Substance Abuse and Mental Health Services Administration (SAMHSA) guidelines.

3. Take note of the oil's CBD concentration
Just like other products in the market, CBD oil can be adulterated or 'watered down.' Some producers seek to maximize their profits by fooling their customers with cheap prices. Customers, in turn, think they are getting a wise bargain while in fact, they have received the fake and not the real products.

It is critical that you pay more attention to the CBD concentration levels too. Quality oil will contain CBD between 250mg to 1000mg per ounce. The concentration levels are critical because if for example, you get a 5-ounce bottle that contains 250 mg CBD, then the concentration will only be 50mg per ounce, which is barely enough to provide you with the full profits of CBD. Therefore, as you search through the market, take note of various concentration levels to ensure that the product you are purchasing can indeed help you.

In the event CBD concentration levels are not indicated, use the following formula to guide your selection:

Divide the total CBD amount by the volume indicated on the container.

For example, divide 1500mg CBD by 4 ounces in for a 4-ounce CBD oil bottle. Each ounce will give you 375mg CBD per ounce.
4. Confirm that the CBD Oil you intend to purchase is pure
From your purchases so far, you certainly know not to take the manufacturers word for it. Manufacturers will always indicate

that their products are free from contaminants.

The sure way to know that your CBD oil is pure is to have it tested at an accredited laboratory, free of the influence of its manufacturers. Laboratories test for the presence of bacteria, heavy metals, fungus, pesticides, foreign material, and residual substances used in the extraction process. If you only want to purchase one bottle, a lab test is a little farfetched. However, you would still be able to assess the purity of your oil from consumer reviews, company reviews, and other sources of objective information.

5. Determine the total amount of CBD in oil
While this may seem redundant and a repeat of an earlier point, it certainly is not. It is also important to evaluate the total amount of CBD you are getting. Most bottles will have the '1000mg CBD oil' label which means that you will be getting 1000mg of CBD from using the entire bottle. Your intended dosage should guide this decision because it determines the interval between your purchases.

6. How was the CBD extracted?
The process of retrieving CBD from the hemp plant is quite complicated. One of the easiest and cheapest methods is to use harsh chemical solvents that leave residues in the oil. However, the best method, which is also the most reliable, uses extremely low temperature, very high pressure, and carbon dioxide to extract the maximum possible amount of uncontaminated CBD. Once the pressure is released, the carbon dioxide simply evaporates and leaves the CBD oil, leaving no traces.

7. Transparency
It is critical that you look out for CBD products that are sold transparently, legally, and with accountability. There are many shady black market businesses with false claims and inferior products. Therefore, finding a transparent company that produces quality products is the first step towards securing your health and ensuring you get the promised outcome.

8. The presence of product claims

The Food and Drug Administration DSHEA has issued guidelines that prohibit the use of medical claims on the effectiveness of CBD products for treatment or to suppression of symptoms. Although initial research has indicated that CBD oil is quite useful for several medical issues, the law indicates that CBD companies should avoid making any direct medical claims. Therefore, in your purchase, beware of companies that disregard this guideline. If a company is willing to defy a simple rule, it is likely that they are defying other product quality guidelines.

9. The Manufacturer's answerability

It is easy for companies to hide under brands and company names, and not release any information about them on the internet. However, you get some relief if the company has listed a genuine phone number that potential consumers can use to reach its people. It is difficult to reach companies selling substandard products and while some may have a get-back-to line, you will be directed to an automated menu that avails no results. Therefore, before making your order, make effort to reach the company. If you are able to reach the company and someone picks the phone or is able to get back to you in a timely fashion, you have found an accountable manufacturer that cares about the quality of its products and the welfare of its consumers.

10. Price Matters

When it comes to purchasing CBD oil, avoid taking cheap options. Cheap does not always mean that the product is a better choice. The process of extracting CBD is not exactly cheap, which means that getting your oil at a low price should make you question the potency, purity, and integrity of the oil. The proper extraction method uses high expertise and complex equipment, unlike cheaper methods that use chemical solvents that leave toxic revenues like ethanol, butane, and propane.

Expensive CBD oil will be that which is organically grown, has a high CBD concentration, and has been extracted using carbon dioxide. It must also have been grown from the United States, made from high-quality plants, tested in quality third-party labs and sold by companies that follow all production laws.

11. Is the CBD Full-Spectrum or not?

The term 'full-spectrum' is used to refer to the entire hemp plant versus isolated parts from which CBD can be extracted. Marketers will often use words like 'all natural' and 'pure' but these do not mean that the CBD was produced from a plant. It could have been synthesized in a laboratory. Although there is much debate surrounding the effectiveness of the full-spectrum CBD, existing research already supports it.

Besides the fact that it causes a person to reap all the benefits of CBD, there is also a keen reason you should opt for full-spectrum CBD — the possibility of contamination. It can be quite an impossible task to trace CBD oil created in the lab back to its producers and the possibility of adulteration and counterfeit production is even higher. Lab-made oils produced overseas are particularly more likely to be contaminated compared to local ones.

If you keenly follow the steps listed above, you are sure to end up with a genuine product.

Chapter 4: How to Dose CBD Oil

Both experienced and first-time users find trouble determining the amount of CBD oil to take. We have already established that legit companies that follow FDA regulations do not have dosage recommendations and will only indicate the amount of CBD in each bottle. The task of determining the amount to take is left to the user.

The CBD oil industry is new and the lack of concrete research has kept the oil manufacturers from making dosage recommendations under the FDA's guidance. This has left consumers estimating their dosages blindly based on recommendations that companies and brands leave behind along with loud disclaimers that the information therein is not verified. Worse still, some consumers get guidance from friends who have used CBD before and claim to be experts.

'A dropper per day' is the most common recommendation out there. However, there is no way to tell whether it is the correct dosage for an individual because it does not account for the individual's weight, body chemistry, the severity of health condition, and the CBD concentration of the oil. This 'one fits all' dosage has left many users on a trial-and-error usage in a bid to determine what work best for them.

Researchers indicate that the receptors in the endocannabinoid system of the body change as the body physiology changes. The endocannabinoid system regulates various functions in the body and if it changes and shifts throughout a person's lifetime, the universal dosage cannot work effectively. How then do you take this incredible oil?

Take up the following simple steps:

1. Follow the direction of your weight
Just as when using many substances, a high body mass requires a higher CBD to feel effectively the effects of using it.

That said, the rule of thumb to determining the right dosage is to take 1mg to 6mg CBD for every 10 pounds body weight, but this is also dependent on the level of pain a person is feeling.

For example, a person who weighs 150lb could take 15mg-25mg while a person weighing 200lb can take 20mg-33mg as a start dose.

The Medium Corporation has come up with a table that you can use to estimate your CBD dosage based on weight and pain levels, from none to severe pain.

	Weight					
Pain	Less 25lbs	26-45lbs	46-85lbs	86-150lbs	151-240lbs	More than 241lbs
None-Mild	4.5mg	6mg	9mg	12mg	18mg	22.5mg
Medium	6mg	9mg	12mg	15mg	22.5mg	30mg
Severe	9mg	12mg	15mg	18mg	27mg	45mg

Table 1.1: Table showing an estimated dosage of the CBD oil based on weight and levels of pain.
CBD oil users can use the table to come up with an estimate of the amount of CBD they need in their CBD oil dosage.

2. *Begin with a small dosage and increase it progressively*
People are created differently and have different histories in regard to the use of supplements, substances, medications, and other elements we take into our bodies. This causes each person to have a unique body chemistry, which in turn determines how the body reacts to different CBD levels. What works for one person may not work for another.

Even for people with the same weight, the CBD dosage should be independent. For example, if a friend weighing 180 pounds takes 22.5mg CBD twice per day and it works well for him, and you weigh the same, do not take up his dosage for yourself too.

Instead, use your unique statistics and observe how your body reacts to different amounts of CBD, beginning with a small dosage, and gradually increase until you have worked out an optimal dosage that produces the benefits you anticipated.

3. Involve your doctor
The third step, one that is highly recommended, is to refer to your physician particularly if you have an existing condition. Not many doctors have had experience working with CBD, but many will have an idea of how your body will react to CBD and will provide professional guidance on the right CBD dosage for your condition.

While you may already know the amount of CBD to take, the task now lies in accurately measuring your CBD dosage. Do you have an idea of the CBD content in a single puff from a vaporizer? Do you know the amount of CBD in a drop from a CBD tincture?

Without a proper understanding of how to measure these dosages, determining the amount of CBD to take in is pointless. However, if you are stuck on this one step, here's how to measure each in line with the method of intake.

Measuring Your CBD Vape Dosage

A CBD cartridge system or a CBD e-liquid system is used to measure vaping CBD. Whichever method you use, the equipment is easy to use and offers an enjoyable experience.

When you use an e-liquid to vape the CBD, start by measuring the amount that is in the dropper. (This method also applies when using a tincture). Once you determine this volume, you will know how much you will be putting into a tank. Vape during the day and keep a close eye on the number of refills you make and the amount of time between them.

For example, if you have determined that the correct dosage for you should be 25mg and you have purchased a 1000mg bottle of CBD oil, one tank should contain approximately 33.33mg CBD. This means that you should only vape one tank by dividing it into smaller amounts. As you can see, this dosage is not 100% accurate but with time, with consistent monitoring, you will establish your optimal CBD intake.

Using A CBD Tincture to Measure Dosage

A CBD tincture makes administering the CBD dosage quite easy. You only need to let the oil into the dropper and place the oil under your tongue for 30-90 seconds before you swallow it. The question now is on the number of CBD oil drops to take. Well, some mathematics will help you come up with a specified plan.

For starters, since you will be using the CBD tincture to measure the amount of CBD in a dropper. A typical dropper holds 1ml of a liquid and when you know the volume that a CBD tincture holds, you can use a simple formula to determine the amount of CBD that is in the dropper.

Here is the formula:

(The total amount of CBD as indicated on the bottle)/ (The number of milliliters in the tincture) = The amount of CBD in a dropper

If, for example, you have a CBD tincture that holds 30ml CBD in a bottle containing 1500mg CBD, you will draw approximately 50mg CBD in every dropper.

1500/30= 50mg CBD per dropper.

Therefore, if your dosage is 25mg CBD and has established that each dropper carries 50mg CBD, you only need to fill the dropper halfway.

Of course, this method too is not definite, but it is better than failing to put in any form of measurement. Remember that for this method too, you will need a small dosage for your initial intake, and with time, you can increase your intake until you determine the optimal dosage.

The Most Accurate Method of Taking CBD Oil

So far, the methods discussed have used estimates based on the tools available for use. However, there exists a more accurate method to take in CBD oil. This method uses CBD capsules.

CBD capsules uniformly contain the same amount of CBD and provide an accurate measure of CBD dosage. If you have established that you will need 16mg-25mg CBD, then you will only need to purchase a bottle of capsules with the 20mg or 25mg CBD concentration. This method is easier than when using a CBD tincture or vape. You only take a capsule and you are good to go for the entire day.

Chapter 5: How to Ingest CBD Oil

While reading about CBD oil dosage in the previous chapter, you probably got clues on the methods of taking this healer liquid. The four primary methods are ingestion, inhalation, sublingual, and topical application. This chapter discusses these methods in depth to get you to be more knowledgeable about the options at your disposal.

Ingestion

This is the most prevalent and common method of taking CBD oil. A person takes in the oil through the mouth, allowing it to pass through the digestive system before it is metabolized in the liver. Once the metabolism is complete, the active compounds produced are sent to the bloodstream to perform various functions such as pain reduction. This is also the method used when taking daily supplements and vitamins.

CBD oil products to be ingested typically come in the form of oil, candy, capsules, beverages like coffee, and other edibles. If the oil taste is uncomfortable, the CBD oil can easily go down with a glass of water. You can also mix it with other items like baked goods, juices, and salad dressings.

Sublingual Option

If you choose the sublingual option, you will place the right amount of CBD oil under your tongue and hold it there for 30-90 seconds before you can swallow it. This time is meant to give the mucous membranes ample time to absorb active ingredients from the oil directly. This administration method is advantageous because the active compounds immediately get into the bloodstream, bypassing the journey through the digestive system and the metabolism process of the liver. This way, the cannabinoid compounds are able to link up with the endocannabinoid system more readily and easily. For those looking for immediate relief, the sublingual option is the most ideal.

The remaining oil then passes down the digestive system and is slowly digested, metabolized, and released into the system. The sublingual method is therefore ideal because it provides both immediate and continuing relief. Persons who adopt this method are mostly those using CBD tinctures, pure CBD oil, and concentrates.

Inhalation

This method is only ideal for adult persons who have encountered vaping before. Getting a non-smoker or a child to learn how to use a vaping pen to inhale the oil is complicated and unnecessary. In this method, the CBD oil is aimed at the lungs where it is absorbed into the bloodstream quickly and then redistributed into the body. This method is also quite fast because the oil bypasses metabolism in the liver.

Although this method is tedious and only reserved for a few, it is considered the most efficient CBD application method because it gets a larger share of the original product into the bloodstream than any other methods used.

CBD meant for inhalation will typically be in the form of a vaporizer e-juice made by infusing CBD oil into a high-CBD concentrate or in vegetable glycerin. The vaporizers themselves will vary in size, from small battery-powered pens to large tabletops and plug-in electric units.

Topical Application

Some manufacturers design their products containing CBD oil for topical application. When CBD oil is taken in through this method, its active compounds are absorbed through the skin where they are able to interact with body cells without getting into the bloodstream. This makes topical application ideal for persons seeking relief from skin conditions because they are applied to the areas they are needed.

Majority of the topical CBD oil products currently on the market are in the form of body care and bath products such as salves, lotions, moisturizers, shampoos, and soaps. These products are designed for daily use to ensure that the skin revitalizes and regains its health.

The CBD oil application forms discussed above are meant to increase choice and options for consumers. They are designed in a manner to make them easy to use and offer fast relief.

Chapter 6: What to Be Careful About, When Ingesting CBD Oil

The safety of using CBD oils among adults has been a subject of research for many small-scale studies in the past and all the tests conducted showed that adults could tolerate a wide range of doses very well. No serious effects on a person's mood, vital signs, or on their central nervous system were reported, even among those that consumed high CBD doses. Only a few said they felt tired or experienced appetite changes, weight changes, and diarrhea, but in general, the oil was found to be a safe product.

That said, it still important to take caution when using CBD oil. There are some claims that CBD oil triggers some side effects like vomiting, drowsiness, nausea, appetite changes, dizziness, anxiety, dry mouth, diarrhea, drowsiness, and mood changes. There is also a concern that taking the CBD oil could overwork the liver by increasing the liver enzyme levels. Increased enzyme levels are a marker for liver inflammation and damage.

Below is a brief description of each documented side effects.

Nausea: Some users have reported experiencing some stomach discomfort after ingesting CBD oil. While this is only based on reports and customer reviews, there is no scientific explanation for it. Indeed, CBD oil is meant to boost a person's appetite and suppress nausea, which makes nausea an unusual side effect. However, those that felt nauseated reported that the feeling was mild and that it went away very quickly. If you feel nauseated too, lower your dosage and you will feel better in no time.

Headaches: While CBD oil is used to treat pain, some people reported that it caused them headaches. Thousands of people have reported experiencing relief from migraines and headaches after consuming CBD oil, which makes the claim that the oil causes headaches more of a mystery. It is likely that those who did indeed have a headache used low-quality CBD oil that still contains contaminant solvents like isopropanol and ethanol, to which some are sensitive. Therefore, if you experience headaches, you should probably try switching to higher-quality hemp CBD oil and you will see that the headaches will go away. It is also important to admit that people have different body chemistries and that if you feel uncomfortable after using CBD oil, perhaps it is not the best fit for you.

Low Blood Pressure: Some people experience a slight drop in their blood pressure when they take very large CBD oil doses. This occurs almost immediately after the active CBD compounds get into the bloodstream. The worst you could expect when this happens is lightheadedness that lasts only for a few minutes. This mainly happens to persons who have had problems with their blood pressure or are in the course of medication for it. Therefore, speak to your doctor before you attempt to use CBD oil because it may not be right for you.

Dry Mouth: CBD oil is likely to cause dry mouth among some users. Research studies conducted are yet to explain this phenomenon but a 2006 study showed that CB1 and CB2 receptors in the body regulate the production of saliva. Therefore, when CBD oil compounds activate the receptors, saliva production reduces and the person experiences dry mouth. Dry mouth is simply having the feeling that your mouth is dry and it will only prompt you to take a little above normal amount of water.

Parkinson's disease patients experience more tremors: People living with Parkinson's disease should consult their doctors before making the decision to try CBD oil. Studies have indicated that when taken in high doses, the oil aggravates the muscle tremors linked to Parkinson's disease. At low doses, this oil is actually quite helpful for patients with the disease. However, because of the ambiguity surrounding safety and dosage of CBD oil, it is only right if persons with the disease visit with their doctor before they try anything.

Dizziness: The dizziness or lightheadedness feeling is often associated with low blood pressure. As mentioned, some people may have this feeling immediately the oil compounds get into their systems. This should pass on its own after a few minutes or you could try to lay down a bit, have a cup of tea or coffee, or even snack on a piece of chocolate. These calming activities offer tremendous relief to your dizziness and blood pressure problem.

Sleepiness: This side effect is no surprise because one of the uses of CBD oil is to put to sleep people suffering from insomnia. In low quantities, CBD oil brings down any anxiety or pain and causes you to relax. However, in large doses, you are bound to fall asleep. If you experience drowsiness when you take CBD oil, at all costs, avoid taking it before doing activities that require attention like driving or operating machinery. Kindly note that it may take a while for the CBD oil to kick in sometimes, and you could quite easily get into trouble if you fall asleep on the job or on the road.

Although research into CBD oil is still in the initial stages, studies conducted so far shows that the oil is safe but for the tiny mishaps mentioned above.

There are also fears that CBD oil could interact with other medications like anti-epileptic drugs. The American journal Pediatrics published an article by the American Academy of Pediatrics (AAP), which cautioned nursing mothers and pregnant women to keep off marijuana because it affects the development of the baby.

A second study conducted to review the accuracy of this AAP report also studied the effects of a short-term exposure to CBD and found that it increases the porousness of the placenta barrier, increasing the chances of the fetus accessing certain dangerous substances from an unhealthy mother.

It is also true that depending on the extraction process, some CBD oils in the market could contain THC. This element impairs your ability to function properly such as the inability to operate machinery or to drive safely, and in the long-term, THC could also affect your mental wellness, attention, heart rate, and mood. It is also quite easy to overdose on the CBD. Therefore, when you decide to take some, begin with a small dose and ensure that you wait awhile because it may take some time for the effects to be fully felt after consumption. Avoid taking another dose.

In lieu of these side effects, both experienced users and those considering taking up CBD oil ought to consult their physicians first of these possible side effects. This does not only apply to pregnant women and nursing mothers but also to other population groups. In one of the studies designed to test the effects of using CBD oil, it was observed that children with conditions like refractory epilepsy who used CBD oil intensified their symptoms. They experienced more aggravated seizures, drowsiness, irritability, and digestion problems. Therefore, people with these problems should not attempt to use CBD oil.

CBD oil is also known to interact with other drugs, especially those that need to be metabolized by the liver. CBD inhibits the working of liver enzymes that break down the pharmaceutical drugs. Once the metabolism process is interrupted, the workings of a drug in the body change too. However, the change or effect that the CBD oil brings to the body is similar to that which would be if you ate a grapefruit, which means that it shouldn't' alarm you much. However, it is still important to check with a doctor before you start taking CBD oil to discuss any likely complications when the oil starts interacting with your medication.

It would please you to know that regular consumption of CBD oil does not present any health concerns. A study conducted in 2006 found that acute administration of CBD does not produce any noteworthy toxic effect in people. This study administered doses of between 10mg to 400mg to healthy volunteer subjects every day for a period of 30 days. At the end of the month, there were no psychiatric, neurological, or clinical alterations to their bodies. A later study also proved this fact when it showed that consuming 1500mg CBD oil per day did not produce any toxic consequence, concluding that the oil is well-tolerated in the body. The two studies also noted that there were no withdrawal symptoms, both for the high and the low dosage, which means that it is impossible for a person to develop chemical reliance on CBD.

The purity of the oil continues to be a matter of concern, however. The Journal of the American Medical Association (JAMA) published a research letter in 2017 after analyzing 84 CBD products drawn from 31 online companies. The research produced startling results, which showed that at least one in five products had intoxicating elements like THC that would be dangerous especially if consumed by children. There have also been reported cases where CBD products contained fungi, fungicides, and herbicides. As the industry grows, we can only hope that there will be stricter regulation and inspection to check the purity levels of most CBD oil products on the market.

Chapter 7: CBD Oil Manufacturers

The much-touted CBD oil is currently available online, in health food stores, grocery stores and at vape shops. People are increasingly aware of the health benefits and many countries and states are rethinking the legality of marijuana and its various products. Regulatory and legal barriers are slowly being lifted and consumers are growing increasingly interested in experiencing the CBD oil benefits for themselves. This sudden explosion of the infant cannabis industry has attracted a number of players in the market who wish to benefit from this much profitable global industry.

With much success comes imitations and fakes, consumers need to be aware of the best brands in the market. As discussed in previous chapters, the effectiveness of your oil and the assurance that you will not be victim to some side effects lies in your ability to acquire a pure product from a reputable producer.

Below is a list of the top CBD oil manufacturers in the world in 2018. This list gives you the option of choosing between local companies and companies abroad, whichever suits your pallet. Check out their names when looking for some of the best CBD oil in the market.

CV Sciences
CV Sciences is a US-based company with its facilities and offices located in San Diego, California, and in Las Vegas, Nevada. CV Sciences, formerly CannaVest, leads in the production and marketing of hemp-based cannabinoids like CBD oil for personal use. It also supplies it to industries like the specialty beverage, beauty care, nutraceuticals, and pet care industry, among others. This year, the company has reported remarkable profitability and success, which is a demonstration of the quality of its products and the level of brand recognition it has achieved in the CBD oil market. CV Sciences' PLusCBD oil product line is well positioned to expand distribution and

for mainstream approval even as the health and wellness authorities continue to embrace the commercialization and standardization of hemp and marijuana-based products. CV Sciences recently raised the number of its retail stores to 1968, making it one of the largest CBD oil distributors in the world.

Gaia Botanicals

Also known as Bluebird Botanicals, Gaia Botanicals is a top award-winning CBD oil producer and is the global leader in the manufacture of Hemp CBD consumer products. Although much of its retail business is done online, the company also has brick-and-mortar retail stores and has also partnered with numerous third-party retailers.

For a while now, Gaia Botanicals has been privately labeling its products for other companies around the world and selling some of its pure CBD extracts to other companies. Because of this, Gaia Botanicals now has a wide reach with distributors in Europe, South America, and Japan. Plans are underway to reach other regions too. Some of the products the company trades include CBD capsules, vape equipment, and fluids, CBD extracts, and other products meant for pets.

Medical Marijuana

Medical Marijuana is a leading company dealing with cannabis-based and industrial hemp products. It produces CBD oil that is used in the manufacture of cosmeceuticals, nutraceuticals, and pharmaceuticals. Medical Marijuana currently operates through its numerous subsidiaries like Red Dice Holdings, HempMeds, HempVap, Wellness Managed Services, CanChew Biotechnologies, Kannaway, Hempwire, and HempMeds Brasil. HempMeds Brasil has already been authorized to sell CBD oil products in Brazil for the treatment of Alzheimer's, multiple sclerosis, and autism spectrum disorder. Medical Marijuana hopes to enlarge its customer base as more governments across the world ease regulations surrounding the use of cannabis and hemp-based products.

CBD American Shaman

CBD American Shaman is famous for producing CBD oil with high CBD concentrations. Its oil is high-quality and the positive reception in the market is clear proof of this fact. The company is now one of the largest in the CBD oil market courtesy of its resolve to shift CBD products from the traditional smoke and vape shops, and the campaigns it has conducted to increase the people's awareness of the benefits of CBD oil.

CBD American Shaman's products are high-quality and unique in a special way because they are extracted from organic naturally grown industrial hemp without contamination from heavy metals, insecticides, and GMO. They are also purely gluten-free.

Some of Shaman's products in the market include skin care products, pain relieving hemp oil, CBD oil tinctures, and feline and canine hemp oil. These products contain rich CBD extracted through the cold pressing method that leaves the oil pure with no contaminants.

Elixinol

Elixinol has made a name for itself as one of the companies that manufacture and produce the highest quality organic hemp products. The company itself is divided into three segments based on location and the kind of products produced. The segments include Elixinol USA that produces dietary supplements, Elixino Australia that produces medicinal cannabis, and Hemp Foods Australia that supplies food products.

Elixino's main production activities remain in its United States location, from where the products are distributed to the United States market, and to consumers in other countries like Japan, the UK, Brazil, and Puerto Rico. Lately, the company has taken up a disciplined approach to pursue growth, which has seen it get into unchartered markets.

Aurora Cannabis

This too is one of the top CBD oil producers in the world. Aurora Cannabis primarily deals with the production and marketing of marijuana products for medical purposes. However, this esteemed company also produces THC and other psychoactive products. Having been quite successful in the market, Aurora is set to be one of the largest CBD oil producers in the world.

Aurora's current resources already allow the company to produce more than 570,000 kg every year and this could increase with time. This capacity to produce large quantities has placed the company at an advantage, to take up any upcoming market and demand as the people increasingly become aware of the benefits and the availability of CBD oil particularly those in the European market. Aurora Cannabis uses its fully-owned company Pedanios to distribute its products and to ensure that they are up to the GMP standards of the EU.

Canopy Growth Corporation

As you would expect, Canopy Growth Corporation also leads in the production of marijuana products. It mainly manufactures them for medical reasons and distributes them through its popular subsidiary Bedrocan. This outsourcing has enabled the company to focus on production only and allowed Bedrocan to charter its ways around the global markets. As of now, it has already penetrated the Brazil and Germany markets.

In the marketplace, Bedrocan is hyped as one of the most experienced producers and distributors of medicinal cannabis in the world, selling products made from five different strains of the cannabis plant.

IRIE CBD

IRIE CBD is a top company producing health and wellness products. It majors on the production of organic high-quality CBD hemp products and selling them to consumers at an affordable price. Its products are exclusively non-GMO and are grown in soils rich in nutrients. The company has a large portfolio of CBD health products that continues to expand year after year.

Isidiol International

The Isidiol International Company has been in the business of providing health and wellness products for a while now, and recently, the company ventured into the production of CBD products. It uses the CBD extract as a source of active pharmaceutical ingredients for their quick and lasting benefits. It is currently running marketing campaigns to get consumers to understand and purchase CBD oil products. These products are sold both in the domestic market and abroad.

Endoca

On a volume basis, Endoca is Europe's largest CBD oil producer. The company has all its major operations situated in the UK, but it also runs an office in the United States. Endoca has indicated that it only makes its products from natural, organic, and certified hemp plants on which herbicides, pesticides, and other chemicals have not been used. As a result, it produces some of the finest CBD oil and other cannabinoids available in the market.

Endoca has taken up control of its entire value chain, from growing to harvesting to processing and marketing. It also has its own warehouse and does its own shipping. The company is now working on a project to channel solar energy for power as its contribution towards environmental conservation. Endoca is surely in charge of every activity that relates to its products to ensure that it delivers quality to consumers in a socially responsible way.

Other companies that produce good quality CBD oil include Plus CBD oil and Beyond Botanicals, both located in the United States.

The future cannot be brighter for these CBD oil-producing companies. The radical growth in popularity of e-commerce over the years and the willingness of customers to make purchases over the internet has promoted online retailing. Online trading supports both business-to-business (B2B) trading and business-to-customer (B2C) trading.

Many of the CBD oil producing companies are turning their attention on these internet savvy customers and are now opening portals and websites to showcase their products to them. This model of business will help CBD oil producing companies reduce their production costs and other overheads, allowing growth and expansion so that more consumers get to experience the wonders of this miraculous oil. They will also reap larger profits.

Chapter 8: Manufacturing Process

This chapter briefly covers the process of extracting and manufacturing CBD oil before packaging it for delivery to consumers.

The extraction process
As mentioned in previous chapters, CBD oil is extracted from the hemp plant in a number of ways, one of them involving the use of liquid CO_2, very low temperatures, and extremely high pressure. However, the first step is to ensure that you have the right plant and that the plant is legal in the market you wish to reach.

The plants to be processed should have high CBD concentrations. Plants that have a high CBD concentration often have low THC levels. Therefore, many manufacturers prefer working with the CBD-rich hemp plant than other members of the cannabis family. Still, CBD levels can also vary among hemp plants and therefore, companies tend to lean towards those that are distinctively potent. The selected plants are harvested from the fields using a combined harvester and transported to the factory for extraction.

1. Extraction Using Chemical Solvents
Once the ideal hemp plants are in the factory, it is time to initiate the extraction process. Some producers use solvents to separate the essential oils from the seeds and the stalks. The liquid is pushed into the now ground hemp material and it dissolves all the lipids, CBD oils, and useful compounds. Some solvents also drain out the chlorophyll, giving the plant a rich green color and a bitter taste. The solvent is then drained out leaving oil that is rich in CBD.

2. Extraction Using Carbon dioxide (CO_2)
The CO_2 extraction method is simple too. It uses temperature and pressure to change the state of matter of carbon dioxide from solid to liquid to gas. The extraction process is done in a

closed-loop extractor. This is a machine with three chambers. The first chamber contains dry ice, solid CO_2. The second chamber has the plant material, while the third chamber carries the final product.

During extraction, the solid carbon dioxide (dry ice) is pumped into the second chamber where it interacts with the plant material. This second chamber has the ideal temperature and pressure to allow the dry ice to become liquid. Running through the material, the liquid Co_2 carries with it elements and flavors just like in the solvent method. The CO_2 cannabinoid mixture is then pumped into the third chamber with an even lower pressure and higher temperature that causes the liquid Co_2 to shift back to a gas state. It rises to the top of the chamber leaving behind the oils to be collected for manufacturing.

The Co_2 method has many advantages. First, it does not take much time for the liquid CO_2 to evaporate as it does when using other liquid forms to extract the CBD oil. Therefore, there is minimal risk, contamination, and interference with the finished product. Second, this method involves pressure and temperature control, which means that it could also be used to separate CBD and THC in the event the hemp plant has high levels of unwanted THC.

3. Olive Oil Extraction

The olive oil extraction method is also one of the most popular extraction methods, but this method is only suitable for small-scale, domestic producers. The CBD in the cannabis plant material fuses with the olive oil creating a CBD and olive oil mixture. This method dates back to biblical times or even earlier, which is proof that it is effective.

First, the plant material is heated for a length of time until it reaches a specific temperature in a process called decarboxylation. Olive oil is then poured in and the mixture is heated to reach a temperature of 100 degrees Celsius. This takes about 1 to 2 hours to provide ample time for the olive oil to extract the CBD. The use of olive oil for extraction makes it difficult to evaporate the solvent, which means that users will have to consume more of it to get their preferred CBD dosage. This oil is also highly perishable and should be stored in a dark cold place. This method is not ideal for commercial producers but it is a simple and inexpensive method suitable for individual consumption.

The three extraction methods discussed above are the most commonly used to extract CBD from the hemp or cannabis plants. Just like marketing channels continue to evolve, it is likely that technology in the CBD extraction process will advance too, paving way for a newer advanced method of CBD extraction in the years to come.

The oil dewaxing process

The extraction process leaves behind fractioned cannabinoids and other extracts that need additional processing. Although these extracts have all the active ingredients that are required in the final product, they need to be refined further before the oil is ready for medical use. At this stage, the extract is raw crude.

The raw crude contains many plant pigments, waxes, and other impurities that are taken out through dewaxing. The dewaxing process begins seeking out a food grade solvent like ethanol to make the undesired waxes separate from the rest of the fluid, based on their solubility and composition, as determined by the extraction process. Taking out these waxes helps to increase the concentration and purity of the cannabinoid.

When you chill the remaining mixture in a freezer, you will find that the waxes begin to separate themselves and you can now dewax the remaining mixture by sieving. This process causes the breakdown of fat, separation, and elimination of waxes from the wintered material. It is important because it causes the cannabinoid liquid to be more stable, in preparation for the formulation process. Dewaxing is also important because it causes the final oil to be more potent. If done correctly, dewaxing should produce separate layers of polar and non-polar substances in the solution.

Dewaxing produces hemp wax. This wax contains only traces, if any, of the cannabinoids. Some producers save the wax for other uses but majority destroy it. The temperature, the time allowed, and the amount of wax in the solution, however, are the determinants of how efficient and safe the process of removing wax is. Each dewaxing process aims to remove all the wax from the solution because the lesser the wax content in the solution, the more potent it is.

Companies dealing with large loads often require multiple dewaxing and filtration exercises with an adequate time allocated between them, to allow the complete and successful precipitation of waxes.

Filtering the CBD oil

The final dewaxing step is filtration. It is done once the waxes are separated and wintered successfully, which happens once the solution has reached a specific temperature. Successful dewaxing separates active from non-active components by removing the wax while keeping the cannabinoids still edged in the solvent. Filtering now removes all the solidified wax out of the solution and preserves the solution which is purely a combination of CBD and the solvent.

The filtration process is done typically using a food grade filtration system in which the supernatant is conveyed to a clean vessel. An expert processing technician decides on the kind of filtration process to use depending on the workability of the solution at hand. Some of the filtration methods include vacuum filtration, wintered filtration, gravity filtration, and pour-through filtration. The aim of either of these methods is to force the chilled solution to pass through 0.2μm porous material and leave behind all manner of waxes.

After making enough attempts to stabilize the temperature of the solution, a sample is drawn to determine whether there could still be some wax remaining in the solution. The success of filtration depends on the equipment available and on the experience of the technician. Filtration is not just a one-time process, it continues through a number of cycles until testing indicates that the liquid has achieved the maximum purity.

Please note that a centrifuge is extremely important in this process because it makes the work even easier. The filtration process can last somewhere between 2 and 5 days depending on the technicians' skills and the efficiency of the available equipment.

Removing the solvent

Once you have gotten rid of the wax completely, it is now time to separate the CBD oil from the solvent. The waxing and filtration processes leave the cannabinoids still suspended in the solvent and now, the solvent needs to be removed.

Solvent removal is done in a special and careful temperature and vacuum control process that is created to prevent degradation of the cannabinoid compounds themselves. Cannabinoids are naturally heat-sensitive and a wrong temperature can quickly adulterate and reduce the strength of the liquid extracted.

Most oil producers use a rotary evaporator for this process. The evaporator is equipped with the right accessories to aid efficient solvent removal. Some of these accessories include a heating bath whose temperature can be adjusted adequately to meet the necessary temperature changes, a vacuum pump, and a bulb mad of the right material and size. Depending on the specifics and the nature of the solvent used, the rotary evaporator is set, being careful to maintain and protect the purity of the cannabinoids present.

If the solvent extraction process is done correctly, the solvent can be recovered with a 90% or greater purity measure and often times, the solvent is reused in future CBD oil extraction processes. This saves the manufacturing company a great deal of money and warehouse expenses associated with bulk solvent purchases.

Many companies find carbon dioxide extraction superior to

ethanol extraction because of the large labor, storage costs, and the price of the solvents used in the extraction and processing stages when using ethanol. Storing and recovery of the highly combustible ethanol at high temperatures also presents a fire or explosion risk that could bring down the entire company.

The distillation process

Even with the highest levels of expertise and care in the previous steps of the CBD oil extraction process, it is impossible to avoid or prevent impurities in the final product. The most skilled and experienced technicians also find it extremely difficult. As such, a final distillation process is needed to come up with a pure form of the extract.
Besides removing impurities, the distillation process also isolates terpenes, a vital element in the making of cannabis medical products. It also purifies and concentrates various cannabinoids, primarily the CBD, and other cannabinoids like CBN, CBG, and CBC among others. Lastly, this final distillation process decarboxylases cannabinoids to make them orally bioavailable.

This final distillation method is referred to as Short Path Distillation. It is the refining process, making it the most important of the distillation steps. It is also the riskiest process and should be handled by an experienced technician. Conducting this process without the right tools and expertise would destroy both the cannabinoids and the terpenes. Therefore, the distillation system is built in a piece-by-piece manner to ensure optimal functionality.

Just as in the solvent extraction distillation process, this one also uses a combination of vacuum, temperature, and circulation controls and manipulations to separate different extracts derived from the cannabis plant. A proper Short Path Distillation process will yield 75% to 90% cannabinoids, but this is all dependent on the technicians' proficiency, the material, and the equipment available. The liquid drawn from the distillation is dubbed the CBD distillate.

Isolating CBD

CBD isolation is meant to separate it from other cannabinoid extracts derived from the hemp plant. A successful isolation process yields 99.5% pre-CBD and it appears a white solid in the form of crystals, granules, and powder. The isolation process takes place in a number of steps that require knowledgeable staff and the right kind of specialized equipment.

The isolation process uses both distillation and chromatography to isolate the CBD, producing an 80-90% pure CBD. At this level of purity, CBD immediately crystallizes forming pure CBD crystals. To remove them from the CBD distillate, the crystals are precipitated from the solvent, which could be supercritical (in the form of both liquid and gas) carbon dioxide or pentane.

Because precipitation of the solvent and chromatography rely on the solvent mixture and recovery methods, getting to the high purity levels requires multiple attempts.

The formulation

Formulation is the process of combining the cannabis extract with different food-grade excipients and carriers to create the final product. The final product is in the form of vape cartridges, capsules, oil, and edibles among many others. Specific calculations are made to determine how much of the CBD extract should be used to reach the intended medicinal strength. For example, CBD to be taken orally will be dissolved into olive oil and a little terpene added to improve the flavor. These combinations, however, must be guided by precise calculations to ensure that the product is safe and will have the expected effect on the product user.

Packaging and labeling

Packaging and labeling prepare the product for transportation to the destined consumer group or market for use. It involves bottling, placing droppers and caps, labeling, and placing the bottles in cartons. All packaging material used must have met FDA standards for food grade items before they are considered for use. The labels on the bottles and on the cartons must have passed through several departments in the company to ensure that the message on them is accurate and that it communicates effectively, to the intended audience. The companies must also be careful to ensure that they do not make any false or illegal claims about the product.

The product testing process

Every CBD oil-producing company has the responsibility of ensuring that the cannabinoid content indicated on the bottle is reliable and that the product itself is safe for consumption before releasing it to the market. Experts test CBD oil by examining it for damage, contamination, and degradation. The primary objective of testing is to ensure that consumers receive the product they bargained for, a high-quality healing oil that will offer relief as promised.

While each producer is free to determine the quality of its products, there are minimum requirements that each product must meet as per the government's federal and local guidelines to ensure that the CBD oil is safe for human consumption. The oil has to pass various tests to check for heavy metals, potency, water activity, pesticide residue, and for the presence of microbial organisms like bacteria, yeast, and mold.

Upon production, all items are held in quarantine until the results of these tests come back. If the products pass each test, the products are released into the market. It is important to note that some local governments place a range around the target amount, such as a +/-5% while others will have exact specifications. Companies also set their own internal specifications guided by the influence they intend to have in the market. This is the reason why some CBD oils in the market will still contain solvents while others will not.

Warehousing

For safety and quality purposes, all plant material, components, materials in process, and the finished products should be stored in controlled environmental conditions. Proper warehousing maintains the integrity of the raw materials and the products so that the manufacturers produce the intended quality of products and for their products to have a consistent quality and taste.

Cannabis and hemp as raw materials should be kept in controlled areas to protect against theft. They should be placed in areas with controlled entry and exit, and the staff manning these areas should be on high alert. Materials that need to be kept under low temperatures ought to be placed in refrigerators.

The raw material in the warehouse should be monitored and tracked by the minute to ensure that all the material is allocated properly when production commences. This means that materials should be organized systematically and carefully in the warehouse, ensuring that all material to be used to make the finished product can be traced.

Distribution

This is the last step on the CBD oil value chain. Companies distribute their finished products according to the size of the markets and other good distribution practices they may have adopted. A proper distribution system is important because it ensures that the right products reach their intended distributors and users.

When handing out the products, the FIFO (first in first out) principal helps to keep the goods in the warehouse in proper rotation. This method ensures that the inventory does not expire while in storage and that it remains fresh, to guarantee the best outcome for users. The FIFO practice also helps to ease distribution because there will only be one batch ready for exit at a time.

All details of the distribution are put down on paper including the batch numbers of the products that are being sent out into the market. This information is critical because in the event there is a recall of the products, each can be traced back to specific shelves and from the end users.

Overall, a good distribution practice helps to maintain a proper seed-to-shelf system.

Chapter 9: Legality in the US, UK, CA, and the Rest of Europe

It is not until recently that countries have begun to legalize cannabis and its products. Many states and countries are still debating whether to allow free use of this plant within their boundaries. This has created variances in the market, and manufacturers and users alike have to conduct a preliminary study of the law to determine if products they wish to distribute or buy are allowed in the specific area. Although CBD is made from the hemp plant and most often will not contain psychoactive compounds, the authorities do not take chances and many that restrict the use of marijuana will often negate the use of CBD oils too.

If you want to know whether recreational marijuana is legal in your neighborhood, it is easy to tell. You will find it in the stores, you can buy it, and the air will tell because the smell will be everywhere. However, it is difficult to tell whether CBD oil is legal. As the purported benefits of CBD oil are increasingly known, stores across the country are stocking the oil on their shelves, vending it online, and you will find it in pet stores too. However, the critical question is – is CBD oil legal?

A closer look at the legal structures surrounding CBD oil use is important because it helps distributors to determine viable markets and also helps consumers to understand the laws, if any, that could restrict their purchases. This chapter, therefore, evaluates CBD oil legality in various major markets around the world.

Legality in the United States

The legality of CBD oil in the United States is quite unclear due to differences in state laws and differences between federal and state laws. This lack of clarity deters many from using CBD oil in fear of being caught on the wrong side of the law. Instead of going on to enjoy CBD benefits, the people are stuck in the lack of knowledge of whether CBD oil is legal.

The fact is that all 50 states allow the use of CBD, but there are still some reservations around it. These reservations differ from state to state, creating divisions between what is and what is not legal. The primary reason for the differences in the legality of CBD and its products is on whether it is derived from marijuana or hemp plants.

The difference between marijuana and hemp plants as mentioned in previous chapters is their THC contents. Marijuana plants contain at least 30% THC while hemp plants only contain 0.3% THC. CBD from the marijuana plant will get a person high but CBD extracted from the hemp plant cannot. Since there is truly no way to determine which plant a manufacturer used, some states have chosen to limit the production and sale of CBD oil altogether.

Therefore, if you ask, "Is CBD oil legal in the United States?" The answer is yes, but only that which contains CBD derived from the hemp plant. The production, sale, and purchase of hemp-based CBD products are entirely legal in the United States. However, the close relationship between marijuana and the hemp plant causes some stigma against hemp-derived CBD.

Marijuana-based CBD products do not enjoy the same privilege. Their CBD is derived from THC-rich marijuana and even if manufacturers work towards eliminating the THC content, marijuana-based products are given the same treatment. Some states allow marijuana-based CBD though, while the rest consider it illegal. These legal indifferences between the states cause much confusion among consumers of CBD products. So, which states allow CBD products for recreational use?

1. States that allow recreational CBD
Only 8 states in the United States have allowed both hemp and marijuana-based products for medicinal and recreational purposes as of 2018. The states include Maine, Colorado,

Oregon, California, Alaska, Nevada, Washington, and Massachusetts. Consumers in these states are free to enjoy any form of CBD without needing a prescription.

2. States that allow Medicinal CBD
So far, 46 states in the United States, counting those listed above, allow medicinal CBD usage but require a prescription. However, despite the fact that all these states allow CBD consumption, the laws in each differ from one state to another. For example, 17 states have restrictions on the amount of THC that a CBD product can have and have restrictions on the health conditions that can be treated using CBD.

The list of these 17 states reads as follows: North Carolina, South Carolina, Kentucky, Alabama, Virginia, Wyoming, Texas, Florida, Georgia, Iowa, Wisconsin, Utah, Indiana, Tennessee, Oklahoma, Missouri, and Mississippi.

The remaining 29 states allow all kinds of CBD products whether derived from the marijuana or the hemp plants. They are Hawaii, Delaware, Arizona, North Dakota, New York, Rhode Island, Massachusetts, Alaska, Florida, Colorado, Michigan, Maryland, Nevada, New Jersey, Pennsylvania, New Mexico, New Hampshire, West Virginia, Connecticut, Arkansas, California, Ohio, Rhode Island, Vermont, Oregon, Minnesota, Illinois, Maine, and Montana. Puerto Rico and Guam territories also allow all forms of CBD products so long as they are consumed on medical grounds.

When purchasing CBD products in the 46 states mentioned above, but for the 8 previously listed, ensure that you get a prescription from a certified doctor. In addition, take precaution and determine the legal THC levels for the particular state in which you are purchasing. States allow having different percentage levels, ranging from 0.3 percent to 8 percent. The legal situation, however, seems to be focusing on the right direction and if you are a CBD consumer in these states, it is important to keep abreast with these changes.

3. States that do not allow CBD and its products

Having listed the 46 states that allow marijuana-based CBD, there are 4 states that adamantly negate the use of marijuana-based CBD. These states are Nebraska, Idaho, South Dakota, and Kansas. Although these states allow hemp-derived CBD, there still lacks clarity on the issue. In this ambiguity, some businesses still sell CBD and patients continue to consume the oil. Persons in these four states should take precaution when using CBD products.

As people increasingly become aware of the benefits of CBD oil, expect that in the next 5 years, all 50 states will have legalized both marijuana and hemp-based CBD oil products. However, with the constantly shifting political environment, it is difficult to make an accurate prediction. Nevertheless, manufacturers and other CBD oil advocates are continuing the campaign, creating awareness of the benefits of CBD.

Legality in the United Kingdom

If you have been keeping a close eye on the last CBD oil news in the United Kingdom, I bet you have realized that now more than ever, people are using CBD oil. The CBD oil market in the United Kingdom has expanded significantly which has led to a nationwide interest in it as people begin to ask what it is and how it benefits the human body. The fact that CBD oil is made from the hemp plant, a cannabis strain, puts to question the legality of CBD oil especially now that there is no clarity on where the United Kingdom stands in regard to cannabis and its use.

For lack of a clear stand on cannabis and its products, the conversation surrounding CBD oil has been divided too. Some believe that it is a legal product while others raise heated opposition saying that it is not. In reality, there has come up full organizations whose primary goal is to push for the legalization of the consumption of CBD oil. Organizations like these are the ones that led to the legalization of CBD oil in 2017. Therefore, today, CBD oil consumption is allowed throughout the nation.

CBD oil was declared legal based on it not being a controlled substance, which means that there is no point of placing any restrictions against its use. Therefore, CBD extracted from any of the 63 industrial hemp plants that the EU has allowed is in turn legal. This law allowing CBD oil into the country has completely transformed the industry for the better, and it looks like this may be the situation for a long time. However, this law does not mean that all kinds of cannabis oils can be used.

While discussing the legality of CBD oil, it is important to take note of an equally important element, THC. In the UK, THC is illegal, which means that there are strict regulations on the amount of THC that can be found in CBD oil. Currently, the UK only allows a maximum of 0.2% THC content, any CBD oil with a higher concentration is illegal, and its use prohibited.

Legality in Canada

On 17 October 2018, Canada became the second country to legalize marijuana on a national scale after Uruguay. Among other detailed aspects of the law was the detail stating that medical marijuana would remain legal, as it has been since 2001. Cannabis oils and parts of the cannabis plants such as the seeds, flowers, and the rest of the plant would be legally sold to consumers. However, cannabis concentrates and edibles would have to wait until 2019 when the law would be reviewed again.

Although cannabinoid oil is legal now, users can only purchase it with a prescription. Patients are only allowed to possess it at their doctors' instructions, which is very important because patients seeking relief from CBD oil are usually dealing with conditions that would be fatal if their drugs interacted with other substances. Therefore, people who wish to purchase CBD oil in Canada should consult their doctors first for a comprehensive evaluation of their suitability to the product's use.

Legality in Other Parts of Europe

Many countries in Europe allow medical cannabis, and by extension, CBD. Countries like Denmark, Spain, Austria, Italy, Belgium, Romania, and the Netherlands are famous for growing medical cannabis and industrial hemp, but only those with none or only about 0.2% THC. Manufacturers across this continent use this industrial hemp in the manufacture of CBD isolates and extracts.

CBD is legal in these countries because it is not placed under the category of controlled substances, and therefore, there are no restrictions surrounding its use. Manufacturers are free to distribute it in their target markets too. However, CBD derived from the cannabis plant is illegal because the law considers the plant itself an illegal drug.

Switzerland has placed unique features in its regulation of the cannabis industry. THC is considered illegal while CBD is legal and can be sold and distributed within the country. However, the country also allows cannabis products that have less than 1% THC, a level significantly higher than that allowed by other countries in Europe. By extension, it also allows its farmers to grow cannabis plants that have a high CBD concentration, so long as they do not exceed the 1% THC value.

Another European country with unique legislation is Luxembourg. Luxembourg has legalized the consumption of cannabis products for medical reasons. In fact, in November 2017, the Minister of Health declared the commencement of a 2-year pilot program that would allow people to purchase medicinal cannabinoids and cannabis extracts to treat various health conditions. This decision was further reinforced in June 2018 when Luxembourg lawmakers approved a bill that proposed the full legalization of cannabis for medical uses. This move allowed more citizens to access medical cannabis to treat or obtain relief from various medical conditions.

The Luxembourg legislations meant CBD product users would have the freedom to use cannabinoids without fear of prosecution. They would also be free to farm cannabis plants provided they only contained 0.3% THC.

Germany too does not restrict the use of CBD oil within its boundaries. The German Narcotics Law does not also list CBD as a controlled substance that needs regulation. However, in 2004, the law was amended to state that citizens would be free to use CBD from the hemp plant only if it did not exceed 0.2% THC.

Many other European countries like the Netherland and France also allow their citizens to consume CBD oil but put restrictions on the maximum THC amount the products should have.

As can be seen in the review of the legality of CBD oil use in various parts of the world, it is clear that CBD is still largely unrecognized and the countries or states that recognize it only allow it to be used for medicinal purposes only. They also clearly indicate the preferred cannabis plant strain and the maximum THC concentration allowed. However, as people around the world become increasingly aware of the benefits of CBD, the laws surrounding CBD oil use are bound to relax a little, to increase the proximity of its products to the people.

Chapter 10: Effects on Anxiety, Depression, and Sleep Disorders

It is likely that at some point, you or a person you know has looked up the internet or asked a doctor for treatment to help with anxiety, sleep disorders, and depression. CBD oils may have come up in the search or the discussion and you wondered how these works. Well, this chapter reviews the use of CBD oils to manage and control anxiety, depression, and sleep disorders.

CBD Oil Effects on Anxiety

A large proportion of the research conducted on marijuana products so far has focused marijuana as a blanket product for all cannabinoids in the market. Many of these studies concluded that cannabis helps relieve anxiety while others say that cannabis products have the capacity to increase a person's anxiety vulnerability. However, this is not the way to get the right information. If you are looking to learn about the effect that CBD oil has on anxiety, focus exclusively on information related to CBD oil, not generalized studies. Although only a few studies have focused on the effectiveness of cannabidiol oil in relieving anxiety, the results of the studies have been promising.

One such study found that using CBD oil significantly reduces social anxiety symptoms among users suffering from social anxiety disorder (SAD). When their brains were scanned, the researchers observed a change in the way blood flows to regions associated with feeling anxious. The study found that CBD oil not only improved the moods of the participants, it also altered their brains' response to anxiety triggers.

In a second study conducted in 2011, researchers sought to address anxiety associated with public speaking. They found that when the subjects used CBD oil, the levels of social anxiety significantly lowered.

The effectiveness of CBD oil was further tested on animal subjects in an identical study conducted in 2014. The results produced were also positive, showing that the oil produced both antidepressant and anti-anxiety effects when applied to animals.

In 2015, researchers conducted an analysis of fragments of research conducted in small-scale studies and found that they all made a similar conclusion. CBD oil showed positive results when used to counter different forms of anxiety such as panic disorder, generalized anxiety disorder, obsessive-compulsive disorder, post-traumatic disorder, and social anxiety disorder. The report, however, observed that not much had been done in regard to studying how anxiety levels change with long-term CBD oil usage. There is research showing that CBD oil offers relief to anxiety on the short term, but none to indicate its effectiveness when used for a long time. Perhaps with increased use and testimonials from consumers, the effectiveness of using the oil to relieve anxiety in the long-term shall be known.

Again, in 2016, a study was conducted to determine whether CBD oil would be useful in reducing post-traumatic stress disorder symptoms for a child that had suffered trauma in the past. The study found that CBD oil significantly lowered the child's anxiety and she could sleep well.

The studies evaluated so far indicate that CBD oil is a powerful remedy for anxiety. So how exactly does it work?

The active compounds in the oil interact with the brain directly. Science explains that CBD lowers action in the amygdala and activates the prefrontal cortex, the two regions of the brains that control anxiety. Some add that it is also able to initiate hippocampus neurogenesis, the process of generating new neurons. This entire process activates CB1 receptors, which positively balance glutamate and gamma-aminobutyric acid (GABA) levels, and hence, CBD is able to reduce anxiety.

Scientists are also hard at work studying possible benefits that CBD could have on persons with bipolar disorder. They are also trying to confirm the anti-psychotic benefits CBD is said to have. Persons with schizophrenia and other mental disorders are reported to experience a reduction of psychotic symptoms after consuming CBD oil.

CBD Oil Effects on Depression

At least one in a group of six people suffers depression all their life. In a year, at least one adult in a group of 15 will suffer depression. These are startling statistics, and the truth is that depression is one of the most incapacitating diseases there are. Sometimes, normal treatment methods only aggravate the symptoms, making the person feel even worse.

CBD oil has been proven an effective solution to a depressed person. While it may not cure the disease itself, it alleviates the symptoms. People who have used it report that they experienced positive results like an improved mood. This is because CBD causes a surge of serotonin levels in the body that causes a person to feel good.

In the treatment of depression, cannabis oil reportedly produces results faster than antidepressants. The active compounds in the oil trigger the endocannabinoid system and speed up the process of growth and development of the nervous tissue, all the while causing little if any side effects.

Cannabis oil is, therefore, a natural remedy that helps patients suffering from depression. It helps them have some peace of mind. They are also able to battle stress better, which improves appetite, enhances the mood, relieves anxiety, battles insomnia, and becomes a source of energy, to enable the patient to have renewed energy and to focus.

A study was conducted in 2006 to examine the effects of daily or occasional CBD oil intake of consumers suffering from depression. The researchers observed that these consumers showed decreased levels of the symptoms of depression compared to those who took alternative treatment methods. A similar study also found that the little THC found in cannabis oil works to improve an individual's response to exasperating situations and emotions by prompting the endocannabinoid system.

Since stress and depression are among the top causes of illnesses, using CBD oil will help alleviate stress, stabilize the mood, and wade off diseases.

To manage depression, consumers should take CBD oil in capsules or in the tincture. They may begin with a small 5mg to 10mg dose and increase the intakes slowly as they begin to observe improved symptoms. Most CBD gel capsules available have a 25mg concentration and since CBD is well tolerated, it is also safe to begin with this dose. Once the CBD is ingested, the effects are felt a few hours later and a person is likely to feel better over the next 24 hours.

If you experience occasional acute flare-ups, the vaporized CBD isolate would be ideal. This method is known to offer the fastest relief and the symptoms die out fast. However, once the emotions have come down, the user should not terminate his dose but should begin taking the CBD either daily or occasionally.

The rule of thumb when taking CBD oil, however, is that a user should consult his doctor first to prevent drugs interacting or the intensification of any underlying medical conditions. Patients are advised to avoid discontinuing or starting any drug in the course of taking CBD without the advice of a physician.

CBD Oil Effect on Sleep Disorders

Since people have been taking CBD oil and other CBD products to bring relief, CBD is now misconstrued as some form of sedative. However, in small doses, CBD is only a mildly alerting compound. It only works like other stimulants such as coffee to activate adenosine receptors in the brain. A number of patients who suffered from sleep issues before have reported that they had a good night's sleep after ingesting the CBD some hours before bedtime.

An alarmingly large population of the United States, approximately 70 million persons, suffer from sleep disorders like insufficient sleep and insomnia among others. CBD proves helpful to persons with sleep difficulties. Some people are unable to sleep because they are anxious and when they take CBD oil, they are able to relax and the quality of their sleep improves. CBD is also said to increase the amount of sleep, which helps patients struggling with insomnia. Some suffer the lack of sleep because of chronic pain and when CBD helps to relieve some of this pain, they are able to sleep comfortably.

CBD not only helps people to sleep, but it also keeps them awake. In small amounts, CBD stimulates the mind to remain alert and rules out drowsiness during the day. An alert mind is able to perform better. Staying awake also strengthens a person's sleep and waking cycle so that he is able to sleep properly during the nighttime.

CBD has a double impact on sleep because it decreases stage three sleep and counteracts sleep the next day. Although THC is known to have a more defined sedative effect, CBD also has a place in sleep treatment. CBD relieves its user from all significant pain and soothes them, leading them to enjoy some sleep. This makes it an excellent element in the treatment of symptoms for people with heart conditions because it eliminates all conditions that would hinder the person's ability to sleep.

Persons with Parkinson's disease can also get relief from their

REM behavior disorder. REM behavior disorder is a condition that causes people to have physical actions as they dream and are in REM sleep. A healthy person's body is in a paralyzed state during REM sleep in a state called REM atonia. The immobilization is what keeps sleeping people from reacting in their dreams. However, a person with REM behavior disorder does not experience any form of paralysis and will move around freely. This disrupts the cycle of sleep and can cause a person to injure himself or other persons sleeping in the room as they move around. CBD helps to improve REM sleep disorders, especially for persons with post-traumatic stress disorder.

Persons with Parkinson's disease also suffer a lot of pain that interferes with the quality of their sleep. However, once they take CBD oil, the pain goes down and the person is able to sleep better.

Some people have found relief from hypersomnolence after consuming CBD oil. Hypersomnolence is a sleep disorder that makes a person acutely sleepy during the day. People with this sleep disorder are inclined to take a nap any time of the day, in whichever kind of environment and they experience no feeling of relief even after they have taken a long sleep during the night or a nap during the day. People with this condition could find relief from CBD because it helps to keep a person alert by stimulating the mind. This way, a person is able to maintain a regular sleep-wake cycle.

Another condition that can be relieved with CBD oil is sleep apnea. Sleep apnea is the condition that causes breathing interruptions for a period of 10 to 30 seconds at a time. Just as it suggests, the lack of breathing could significantly affect the quality of sleep because it interrupts oxygen flow in the body. However, taking CBD oil offers significant relief. Frontiers in Psychology published a study they had conducted to investigate the use of medical cannabis products in treating sleep apnea disorder. Although the medical cannabis was synthetic, it helped reduce the patients' sleep apnea significantly in the short-term and did not affect his sleep architecture. If a synthetic cannabis product was able to offer relief of such magnitude, it is likely that the organic, natural, and rich CBD oil will offer profound benefits to persons with sleep apnea.

Restless leg syndrome is also a sleep disorder whose patients have found relief after consuming CBD oil. As the name suggests, the disorder manifests itself as an irresistible urge to move the legs. This urge increases particularly when a patient is resting while lying down or sitting. This disorder is potentially very disruptive and detrimental to a person seeking to have a peaceful night and quality sleep. Although only a little research has been conducted to study the effects that cannabis has on the restless leg syndrome, the few that has been done has shown positive results.

For example, Sleep Medicine published a study it conducted recently and found that medical cannabis effectively resolved restless leg syndrome in six different cases. The results from this research are not enough to generalize results but as research continues, we are bound to understand how these six patients experienced relief. However, it is clear that the active cannabis compounds largely contributed to the patients' relief.

CBD is able to perform all these sleep miracles by manipulating some functions in the brain. It controls waking by activating some neurons in the DRD and the hypothalamus. Both regions of the brain are responsible for keeping a person alert. This may appear to be counterproductive given that people such as those who suffer from a lack of sleep are trying to increase their hours of sleep. However, CBD's ability to reduce excessive sleeping during the day is what makes it an excellent solution to a person trying to avoid sleep during the day and to have a healthier and longer sleep during the day.

The advantage is that CBD is non-psychoactive which means that it has little if any influence on your bodily functions. This way, a person is able to acquire all the therapeutic cannabis benefits without having to endure unwanted dangerous and disruptive psychoactive effects.

Chapter 11: Effects on Pain, Ailments, and various Diseases (Arthritis, Diabetes, Heart Conditions, and Cancer)

CBD oil is an effective remedy for pain and inflammation, which makes it an effective aid in the treatment and prevention of diseases like arthritis, diabetes, cardiovascular diseases, and various kinds of cancers. This chapter provides a detailed explanation of the CBD's works in each of these conditions.

CBD Oil Effects on Pain

The use of marijuana to treat pain dates back to 2900 B.C. However, it is only now that scientists have focused on the pain-relieving properties of the cannabinoid oil.

One of the reasons driving CBD's popularity is the effect it has on pain. As the USA joins other countries across the world to fight the opioid epidemic that has brought approximately 50 million Americans under the mercy of pharmaceutical drugs, CBD oil seems to be the God-sent alternative. CBD oil is non-addictive and produces little to no side effects. It also offers a selection of ways to use it so that the consumer is able to choose what they find easy and comfortable to use.

The number of persons visiting physicians every day for pain-related issues is quite high and continues to increase by the day. It almost seems like everyone has to suffer from some form of chronic pain at a point in life. While it may prove difficult to predict and to avoid pain, it is promising to see that with proper care and the right products, pain can be treated successfully using natural CBD oil.

By looking at the symptoms of a disease, it is possible to know if CBD will be useful in any way. For example, fibromyalgia patients report a number of symptoms that CBD oil typically addresses. They report sleep problems, chronic pain, depression, anxiety, inflammation, mood issues, muscle spasms, and general mental health problems. CBD oil is known to address the majority of these conditions effectively. Hence, with a doctor's guidance, it is worth trying the oil out.

That said, everyone has unique body chemistry and you will find some singing CBD oil praises while others will say that oil does nothing to improve their symptoms. It is also important to note that different CBD oils contain different CBD concentrations, which could explain why some patients report that they did not note any changes. So far, CBD oil has worked wonders for its larger proportion of users, and it would be bad if you missed these advantages. Get yourself a quality bottle and see if the oil changes anything yet.

As mentioned briefly in the chapters above, CBD works by influencing the endocannabinoid system (ECS), which influences functions like pain, sleep, and responses of the immune system. The ECS already has its own natural cannabinoid, but the addition of CBD increases its functioning because it provides additional exogenous cannabinoids.

The human body has receptors that have a high gravitational effect to cannabinoids and when the exogenous cannabinoids attach themselves to the receptors, they produce an anti-inflammatory and pain-relieving effect. This relaxes the body's immune system, which becomes overactive when a person is in pain. Therefore, taking in CBD produces a calming and soothing effect on the body internally, causing it to relax. Studies have shown that this is what makes CBD an excellent substance to be used in the treatment of chronic pain that is caused by serious conditions like cancer and multiple Sclerosis as will be discussed later in the coming chapters. It is important to note that although CBD relieves pain, it is in no way a cure, and patients should continue to visit their doctors to treat their conditions.

Doctors who deal with the management of pain try to explain the pain-relieving phenomenon by explaining that it is likely that CBD interrupts pain impulses and prevents them from reaching the brain. The Journal of Experimental Medicine published a study suggesting that when CBD oil interacts with receptors of the immune system, it causes an anti-inflammatory effect, which is key to relieving some forms of chronic pain.

Another study seeking to explain this phenomenon wrote that it is likely that the CBD compounds work to prevent the absorption of anandamide from the blood. Anandamide is a pain regulation compound and the higher its concentration in the blood, the lesser the pain a person feels.

The best part of all about using CBD oil is that patients do not become tolerant of it. This is unlike many of the pharmaceutical drugs in the market for whom the body becomes tolerant and the patient has to keep upping the dose or looking for something stronger in the market to get the desired relief. CBD oil is consistently effective and the patient does not develop an addition to it. It is, therefore, a safer and more effective opioid alternative.

How to Treat Pain Using CBD Oil

When coming up with a CBD schedule to treat pain, understand that the CBD oil should be used regularly for it to produce maximum relief. This means that it should be able to prevent the pain before it is used to bring down the pain when it flares up. To do this effectively, only think of CBD oil as a dietary supplement and not a drug so that you are comfortable taking it every day, thereby ensuring that there is a constant baseline concentration of it in your system.

The Benefits

One of the primary advantages of using CBD oil is that it does not produce any adverse side effects. Although a person could feel slightly drowsy and not be able to give maximum concentration when conducting tasks like driving, the sleepiness disappears after only a little while. This side effect is nothing compared to others produced by pain medications. The drowsiness should not be of concern to the users. Instead, they should focus on the benefits of managing their chronic pain and returning to their happy lives as soon as possible.

It is also of great advantage that CBD is well-tolerated. This gives it an advantage over other pharmaceuticals available for pain treatment. Patients have had to choose between anticonvulsants, steroids, opioids, and non-steroidal anti-inflammatory drugs, and all these options produce negative consequences on the people, affecting their health, comfort, and well-being. CBD is, therefore, a positive addition to the group because it does not produce any adverse reaction.

Another top-ranking benefit of using CBD oil for pain is that it does not produce any psychoactive outcome. It does not make its users high. This means that patients of all ages can use the cannabidiol without risking a 'high' and which is one of the primary reasons many patients are now opting for CBD oil. Society is also slowly warming up to the fact that CBD oil is a harmless drug that could help all people with all kinds of pain relief.

CBD is also of benefit because of its capacity to provide relief for other conditions besides pain. As we have already seen, people with sleep disorders, depression, and anxiety also enjoy relief after consuming CBD oil. It is also a mood booster and as we shall find out, it is used for more serious conditions like heart disease. CBD is, therefore, a broad-spectrum aide.

It is impossible to overlook the fact that CBD oil is a natural product. Unlike other medications like opioids that are produced and modified synthetically and will contain all kinds of intoxicating ingredients, CBD is derived directly from a plant. The plants are grown naturally without any pesticides, fungicides, and other elements that would contaminate it. It cannot really get better than that.

Lastly, CBD is relatively cheap compared to prescription drugs. It is cheap in that consumers do not have to spend money repeatedly and that they actually enjoy the desired relief after consumption. Prescription drugs are expensive, seeing that American consumers spend more than $300 billion per year in their purchase. What's more, the drugs do not provide the desired relief and a consumer has to keep revisiting the counters for refills and to see whether the companies have produced something stronger. CBD oil's lasting effects makes it a cheaper option compared to prescription drugs.

In conclusion, the use of CBD oil for pain relief is showing incredible promise in terms of its effectiveness and its increasing awareness among the population. Using CBD to treat pain is now thought to be trendy and it is quickly gaining recognition as a legitimate medical solution. However, the doctor's opinion is still the primary determinant of whether or not you are cleared to use the oil and to ensure that you get the right dosage so that you do not expose yourself to unnecessary risks.

CBD Oil Effects on Arthritis

The Arthritis Foundation says that so far, more than 54 million American adults and about 300,000 children have been diagnosed with arthritis or some other rheumatic disease. In fact, arthritis remains the leading cause of disability among the people. If you add the number of those who have not been clinically diagnosed to the 54 million number, the Arthritis foundation predicts that the numbers could get as high as 91.2 million. The Foundation also expects that the number of people with arthritis will increase by 49% by 2040.

The most common arthritis types are osteoarthritis and rheumatoid arthritis. Osteoarthritis is a progressive disease that affects the bones and joint cartilages, causing stiffness and pain. It mostly affects joints at the thumbs, hip, and knees. Rheumatoid arthritis, on the other hand, is an autoimmune disease meaning that a person's immune system attacks the joints causing inflammation. This form of arthritis primarily affects the feet and the hands causing swelling, pain, and stiffness at the joints.

Arthritis is associated with devastating and dangerous symptoms like stiffness, pain, and decreased joint movement, all of which worsen and intensify with time. Anxiety and depression are also linked to arthritis. It can also become agonizingly difficult to cope with arthritis when a person also has to manage serious conditions like diabetes, heart disease, and obesity.

Studies conducted using animal subjects confirm the word on the street, that CBD can help to relieve patients of the associated arthritis pain and eventually treat arthritis. One such study was conducted in 2011 and the researcher concluded that CBD lowered inflammatory pain in the rat by adjusting the response that pain receptors gave to stimuli. A second study was done in 2014 to review the body of existing studies so far made the same conclusions, that CBD would be effective for the treatment of osteoarthritis. In 2016, another study found that applying CBD oil on the skill relieved pain and inflammation caused by arthritis. A fourth study conducted in 2017 also concluded that CBD oil was a useful and safe treatment that would cure osteoarthritis joint pain.

There is yet to be a scientific study that dealt with human beings to prove the effectiveness of CBD in the treatment of arthritis. However, an earlier study conducted in 2006 had found that Sativex, a cannabis-based mouth spray helped to reduce arthritis pain. However, on testing the contents of the spray in the lab, scientists found that the spray contained both THC and CBD, which prevented them from concluding that CBD alone could relieve arthritis pain. More research using human subjects would greatly help to provide scientific proof of the benefits of CBD oil. That said, people on the ground are continuing to purchase and use CBD oil to treat their arthritis and the results so far have been reassuring.

How It Works

In relieving arthritis pain, the working of CBD in the brain is quite simple. Once CBD gets into the brain, it interacts with CB1 and CB2 receptors to influence pain and the effects of inflammation on the human body. CB2 particularly influences the immune system. Rheumatoid arthritis, on the other hand, causes the immune system to attack the body's tissues in the joints instead of protecting them. The influence of both the CB2 receptor and the rheumatoid arthritis is the reason CBD works well in alleviating rheumatoid arthritis symptoms. CBD's anti-inflammatory properties also help to stop or to slow the advancement of rheumatoid arthritis, to prevent your joints from getting permanent damage. Other arthritis symptoms like fever and fatigue are also addressed.

When using CBD oil for arthritis, both the capsule and the liquid forms work well. Apply the liquid CBD oil onto the skin to help especially in areas with stiff and achy joints. If you choose to take it orally, swallow the capsule and if you are using liquid CBD, add some to your water or food.

Your doctor should be able to help you come up with the right dosage. He will ask you to start small and with time, increase your dosage to an optimum level. Always ensure that you buy the oil from a trusted manufacturer, especially one that provides a full list of the oil's properties.

Effects of CBD Oil on Diabetes

More than 100 adults in America, which makes about a third of the entire population, are living with either Type 1 or Type 2 diabetes. An additional 84.1 million are pre-diabetic and many of them end up with Type 2 diabetes in a span of 5 years only if they do not take precaution. Taking into consideration the fact that these are only clinically diagnosed cases, diabetes is clearly a serious problem in the United States. The situation is also replicated in many other countries across the world, owing to lifestyle changes as the economy improves.

Researchers and doctors are hard at work trying to come up with a situation that could resolve the diabetes issue and luckily, they have stumbled upon CBD oil and other CBD-based products as possible solutions. They sought to determine whether there could be a link between CBD oil and prevention or treatment of diabetes.

The results of the studies have been overwhelming. The scientists have found that indeed CBD oil is useful for preventing and treating diabetes.

One of the best ways of fighting a disease is by preventing it from occurring in the first place. People who are likely to have a positive diabetes diagnosis are those that have high fasting insulin levels or those that have developed insulin resistance. They also tend to have low levels of the high-density lipoprotein cholesterol.

When subjects of a study who used hemp or cannabis regularly were tested on a regular basis over a five-year span, their fasting insulin levels were 16% lower than that of those who did not use any cannabis. This group also had higher lipoprotein cholesterol levels and their insulin resistance levels were found to be 17% lower than those who did not use any cannabis. The study also found that subjects who had used hemp or cannabis in the past but were not current users reported better cholesterol levels, better fasting insulin, and that their insulin resistance was significantly lower than that of subjects who had not used it. However, their results were not as impressive as those of active users were.

One of the facts that came out of this study is that CBD remedies insulin resistance. When the body begins to resist insulin produced in the pancreas to control sugar levels in the blood, the cells of the body cannot absorb the sugar they need to provide energy. This glucose builds up in the circulatory system leading to high toxic sugar levels in the blood. Insulin resistance quickly leads a person to become pre-diabetic or to develop type 2 diabetes.

How It Works

Science does not give a clear explanation of how CBD works in the body to treat insulin resistance, but most researchers credit this ability to its anti-inflammatory capabilities. Many tests done on persons with insulin resistance always bring up chronic inflammation. It is believed that once the CBD is able to lower the inflammation, the cardiovascular and immune systems are able to function better. Sugar metabolism and cell growth also significantly improve when the inflammation goes down. If all body systems are working as efficiently as can be, then the chances of becoming insulin resistant and diabetic by extension, lower significantly.

CBD is also known to prevent obesity, a precursor of type 2 diabetes. Becoming obese and having a large waist circumference increase the possibilities of a person developing diabetes in the future. However, research shows that hemp and cannabis use has a direct relationship with a lower BMI, a smaller waist circumference and lower obesity levels. This is because CBD is involved in several body functions that have weight management benefits. Diabetic persons are able to shed off excess weight brought by inflammation. Obese people are able to stop overeating and therefore stop gaining weight because CBD is an appetite suppressant.

CBD is also involved in an important function that involves fat in the body called fat browning. This is the process by which white adipose fat is transformed into brown adipose fat. Brown adipose enhances the energy burning capabilities of the body while white adipose only stores energy in the form of fats and calories. Therefore, CBD is of great help to persons seeking to lower their weight, to ward off diseases.

GW Pharmaceuticals, a company based in the UK, is currently working on developing a cannabis-based drug that will eliminate the need for patients to have insulin shots to control their blood sugar. This same company developed the cannabis oral spray called Savitex a while ago. Savitex was meant to help reduce the intensity and eventually stop muscle spasms of patients with multiple sclerosis. However, the new drug will be composed of THCV and CBD compounds and will be used to improve insulin production in the body, hence lowering blood sugar.

Tetrahydrocannabivarin (THCV) is also a member of the cannabinoid family that has medicinal value. It has been found useful in bringing a number of health benefits to patients with diabetes such as through suppressing their appetites, which means that it is able to alter the weight of obese people, helping them avoid diabetes.
The American Diabetes Association published a scientific study that had been conducted to look into the safety and efficiency of a combination of CBD and THCV on Type 2 diabetes patients. The researchers found that this combination led to a significant decrease in the fasting plasma glucose and found that the two compounds could be used for glycemic control in patients living with type 2 diabetes.

CBD oil also helps with nerve damage for diabetics. People with diabetes often suffer from neuropathy or nerve damage. Many complain saying that they have lost feeling in their feet or hands or both. However, nerve damage can occur on any organ in the body. This can be detected by pain and some tingling sensations in the areas affected.

In a positive twist, CBD is proving more useful than conventional medicine in dealing with neuropathy. Research shows that it helps relieve pain and prevents damage of the existing nerves. It prevents the liver from going through oxidative stress, which is also a leading cause of nerve damage.

CBD also addresses the negative effects that diabetes has on a person's vision. Diabetes affects vision because the increasingly high oxidative stress in a diabetic can lead to neurotoxicity and an eventual retinopathy, which is simply the loss of vision. However, the active chemical compounds in CBD oil shield the retinal cells and nerves from damaging toxins. The shielding prevents the destruction of the blood-retina barrier, protecting and improving diabetic persons' sight.

The benefits of CBD oil in the treatment of diabetes are summarized as:

- Improves blood circulation by keeping the vessels open
- Evens out blood sugar in the body
- Provides anti-inflammatory benefits that help reduce arterial inflammation that many diabetics suffer from
- Reduces blood pressure gradually, which is of much benefit to diabetic patients
- Calms restless legs, a common condition among people with diabetes
- Using CBD oil instead of regular oil in foods could significantly lower cholesterol in the blood, which is good for the circulatory system
- Relieves and reduces gastrointestinal disorders and muscle cramping with its anti-spasmodic properties
- Reduces chronic pain associated with nerve inflammation by activating receptors in the body
- Prevents complications associated with diabetes like atherosclerosis (plaque buildup in the arteries)
- Protects the optic nerves by reducing neurotoxicity
- Improves a person's glucose tolerance, insulin production, and the sensitivity to insulin
- CBD also acts as a neuroprotectant and prevent nerve damage that sometimes causes diabetic patients to suffer through amputation of their lower body parts.

Overall, CBD is the God-sent miracle to help in the prevention and management of diabetes.

In conclusion, the rise of CBD as a possible natural suppressant of the symptoms and effects of diabetes has been transformative both in the medical field and in the lives of people. It will significantly improve the lives of those who have diabetes and slow down the rate at which people acquire it.

CBD Oil Effects on Heart Conditions

By now CBD oil is coming up as the medical gift that keeps giving because of a large number of benefits it brings to the human body. This section adds to the list if benefits by discussing the therapeutic effect of CBD oil on cardiovascular conditions. Its effectiveness in the cardiovascular system is courtesy of its anti-inflammatory characteristics and the capacity to lower blood pressure.

The cardiovascular system is made up of the heart, blood vessels, and the lungs. These components play one of the most critical physiological roles in the body. The system transports hormones, nutrients, and oxygen to cells in the body, with blood as the carrier agent. Waste products like nitrogenous waste and carbon dioxide are transported out of the system in the same way.

Since the cardiovascular system plays such an important role, it is certain that any form of malfunction or illness in the system has catastrophic consequences. This is the reason cardiovascular diseases are now among the most prevalent causes of death. People die of conditions like coronary heart disease, rheumatic heart diseases, stroke, hypertension and other diseases affecting blood vessels.

Cardiovascular diseases are primarily lifestyle diseases, which is to say that a lifestyle change to include healthy foods and regular exercise could effectively prevent them from occurring. However, another solution is now coming up, courtesy of the cannabis plant. Cannabidiol oil is gaining recognition as an effective therapeutic agent for a number of these cardiovascular conditions.

CBD Oil for a Healthy Heart

You have already learned that the CBD compound in CBD oil does wonders towards the treatment of people suffering from heart-related conditions, but how does it do that? Here's how:

First, CBD strengthens the walls of the arteries. The arteries are like major highways in the circulatory system, which means that they handle the bulk of the oxygenated blood carrying what is needed by the body. This constant passage makes the arteries prone to degradation, especially if the blood is flowing at an unusually high pressure. However, according to a study published by the British Journal of Clinical Pharmacology, taking CBD causes the circulatory system to relax, which reduces vascular tension and preserves the integrity of the artery walls.

CBD also reduces the inflammation of heart muscles. As mentioned previously, CBD interacts with CB2 receptors and enhances the production of adenosine. In other words, when CB2 interacts with CBD, the body's anti-inflammatory chemicals are produced and are able to work better. When CBD interacts with the A2A receptor, inflammation all over the body subsides too.

These anti-inflammatory effects are especially important to persons battling heart disease because the heart muscles swell and when this happens, the person is prone to other kinds of heart ailments.

Another advantage of CBD to the cardiovascular system is that it helps to maintain blood pressure. The Heart Foundation states that high blood pressure is one of the leading causes of heart disease because it increasingly strains the heart and exerts unnecessary pressure on the vessel walls.

In a particular study, patients were handed a placebo or a high CBD dose and their heart rates and blood pressure monitored in a number of ways. The results showed that patients who took CBD experienced a reduced resting blood pressure and a corresponding low blood pressure. The results of this test show that CBD markedly affects blood pressure courtesy of its ability to relax the blood vessels. It causes the arteries t to become less stressed and less tense and from there, the blood exerts little if any pressure on the artery walls, which maintains the integrity and strength of muscles in the heart and the arteries.

One researcher recommended a daily CBD dose to patients who suffer from high blood pressure while another study recommended that all persons take CBD as a precaution against high blood pressure.

In the case of hypertension, CBD suppresses cardiac contractions while helping the blood pressure return to normal, having eliminated the risk of another attack. Therefore, CBD can also be used as a preventative and a treatment option for persons with hypertension.

CBD Oil Effects on Cancer

Scientists are convinced that a combination of both THC and CBD produces one of the most powerful oppositions against tumor growth. CBD is a known anti-cancer element because it is able to interrupt communication between cells in the tumor, as well as its ability to initiate apoptosis, which is the programmed death of cancer cells. Studies conducted by the California Pacific Medical Center, both animal-based and in vitro trials, showed that CBD also affects genes that cause aggressive metastasis by shutting down cell growth receptors.

On the other hand, THC also reduces tumor growth and affects the metastasis rate, even on non-small cell lung cancer, which has become the primary cause of cancer deaths across the globe.

A number of studies have been carried out to determine the effect that a combination of THC and CBD has on brain, cervical, colon, lung, prostate, pancreatic, blood-based, bladder, liver, and other forms of cancer. The studies have found that there is increasing evidence that the two cannabinoids are powerful 'chemo' agents. They specifically target tumor cells and do not leave behind any toxicity on the normal cells. This is unlike standard chemotherapy, which deals equally with a cell on its path, both tumoral and non-tumoral cells.

Besides attacking cancer itself, CBD lessens cancer symptoms and the side effects of treatment like pain, nausea, and vomiting. A study was conducted to confirm this claim. It studied the effect that CBD and THC would have on a sample population of 177 cancer patients experiencing cancer-related pain and symptoms. These people did not find any relief from conventional pain medication.

Study subjects who were treated with a combination of both compounds reported a significant pain reduction compared to those who only took THC. This study proved the pain-relieving quality of CBD, even against chronic pain from cancer.

CBD also helps settle nausea and vomiting that patients suffer after chemotherapy sessions. Although patients are given drugs to help lessen these symptoms, some are ineffective or the patients have become tolerant of them, and are forced to seek alternative medicine.

A study examined 16 subjects taking chemotherapy treatment and found that administering a CBD and THC combination via a mouth spray reduced nausea and vomiting better than conventional drugs did. Added to the fact that CBD causes the death of cancer cells, the CBD and THC option makes patients feel better overall.
Below is a summary of CBD benefits to cancer patients.

- Guards the immune system
- Takes out the repetitive and tiresome pharmaceutical protocols
- Reduces nausea
- Stimulates an appetite

- Increases the possibility of remission significantly
- Reduces or eliminates the growth of malignant cells
- Reduces and eliminates chronic pain

As can be seen in the summary above, CBD is an all-around cancer medication. Although it is not a definite cure for cancer, it lessens the effects of medication and prevents further growth of the malignant cells. CBD oil takes care of the symptoms, making the treatment more bearable.

Chapter 12: Effects on Acne

Cannabidiol, CBD, has found its place in the beauty industry after successfully infiltrating majority of the industries from the manufacturing to the body care industries. Again, CBD is bringing a solution to one of the most prevalent skin problems — acne.

Previously, acne was thought to be a teenage thing and that once the adolescent years were over, the skin would get back to its previous norm and life would continue seamlessly. However, we now know better because acne is common even among adults. Some babies get acne too. The annoying thing is that acne appears in different areas of the body. A person has to tolerate marks and pimples in different parts of the body. Sadly, this constant struggle against acne can be a source of low self-esteem especially when it appears in areas people can see and is persistent.

It is interesting to find out that acne does not only refer to pimples — it is, in fact, an umbrella term and covers everything from cysts, blackheads, nodules, whiteheads, and papules. All these conditions appear when pores on the skin become clogged with waste from dead cells. Bacteria play a role too because it causes the skin to swell and become red.

Acne is caused both by controllable factors and others you cannot control. It is caused by medications, hormones, and diet, particularly that which contains a lot of carbs and dairy products. Some people add stress to the list but stress does not in itself cause acne, it only increases the production of cortisol. Cortisol encourages the skin to release oil that accumulates to form pimples.

The areas of your body that acne occurs the most have the largest number of sebaceous glands and if the glands are connected to hair follicles, upon the release of excess oil, the follicles clog too. A clogged follicle that is plugged causes a whitehead while an unplugged clogged follicle causes a blackhead. These follicles are filled with oil and bacteria that begin to brown and have a dark appearance when exposed to the air. This is how blackheads get their color. Clogged hair follicles can also develop into cysts and pimples.

Some people advocate for waiting until acne fades out by itself, but medical professionals sharply disagree with this idea. This is because if acne is not treated, it scars the skin and leaves dark unappealing spots. These marks can be a source of stress, depression, and low self-esteem.

Acne Can Get Worse

Hormones, medication, stress, and diet trigger the appearance of acne and also make it worse. For example, excessive production of the hormone androgen increases acne, particularly in puberty because it causes oil glands to increase in size, which increases the production of oil, also called sebum.

Interestingly, although overproduction of androgen causes acne, underproduction, particularly among women leads to acne as well.

Pregnancy and birth control also cause hormonal changes that could worsen acne. Some medications, such as those that contain testosterone, corticosteroids (elements used to counter allergic reactions), and lithium increase acne breakouts.

Although people believe that eating greasy food leads to acne, this idea is highly misconstrued. Although diet plays an important part in determining the appearance of the skin, foods contain high carbohydrate levels are the ones that cause or increase the appearance of acne.

Sadly, chocolate also increases acne, although the reason for this is yet to be determined.

Lastly, although we mentioned that stress does not cause acne, it can worsen the situation.

Pharmacies are filled with over-the-counter medications to treat acne. Some people also turn to traditional healing methods. However, CBD is growing as an alternative to all these treatment methods. It has a wide spectrum of benefits for users besides treating acne and it does not cause any major side effects.

Using CBD Oil for Acne Treatment

Just like other body organs, the skin also has CB1 and CB2 receptors that stimulate the nervous system and causes it to work on different functions such as reducing inflammation. CBD oil's anti-inflammatory properties cause a reduction of visible inflammations on the skin thereby reducing the appearance of pimples.

CBD also treats acne in other ways besides reducing inflammation. In one way, it stimulates the endocannabinoid system, which is responsible for cell regeneration. If the regeneration system is not balanced, the skin will be affected in a negative way. Overproduction causes the pores and the hair follicles to clog easily which increases acne. Underproduction has the same effect too. CBD works to restore a balance in this system.

The effect that CBD has on the endocannabinoid system was confirmed in a scientific study. A Hungarian scientist also conducted a study in 2010 to analyze the effect that CBD oil has on the skin. He took up some skin cells and applied CBD to them to see how the oil would react with the body's natural endocannabinoids. The results of the study showed that endocannabinoid cells largely determine the amount of oil that the skin produces. When the body experiences an anandamide surge, it produces more oil. On the other hand, when anandamide levels are low, the skin becomes dry and contracts diseases like eczema. However, when the scientist applied CBD to the human skin cells, anandamide levels went down and the production of oil stopped. This observation justifies the use of

CBD for adults whose skin produces too much sebum making the skin to become very oily. CBD effectively brings down the overproduction and hence there is no extra oil to clog the skin pores.

There are also studies, which have tested the effectiveness of CBD in regulating different skin functions in order to prevent or control acne. The Journal of Clinical Investigation, for example, conducted a study in liaison with the National Institute of Health and they found out that CBD has anti-proliferative and skin regeneration properties. The study was based on the assumption that sebaceous glands on the skin absorb CBD. The sebaceous glands secrete sebum, the oily component that blocks the pores. The researchers found that the CBD on the skin was acting as a sebostatic agent. It reduced sebum excretion, reduced pore blockage, and prevented or reduced acne.

The Federation of American Societies for Experimental Biology also conducted a similar test and got like findings. The study concluded that cannabinoids act on oily skin products and are therefore important for helping the skin maintain a balance between protecting itself against blemishes while preventing dryness. The study also found that CBD may also contain anti-aging elements and that it can be used to treat serious skin conditions like psoriasis and dermatitis.

A study conducted by the National Center for Biotechnology Information in 2014 found evidence to show that CBD has elements that control oil production and thus will effectively control possible skin breakouts. Its use is anticipated to make life easier because many people will cut their doctors' appointments since CBD will act both as a preventative solution and as a treatment solution.

Another study designed to look into CBD and its influence on the appearance of skin using a clinical procedure. The researchers were surprised to find that all their test subjects had visible improvement after only 14 days of use. These results were extraordinary. It is extremely unusual for studies to have a 100% success rate, even when dealing with small samples. However, this particular study showed that CBD oil produced the expected positive results for all participants. This success is another stamp of approval and confirmation on the benefits of CBD in regards to the skin.

People who have tried a variety of acne treatments without much success or that the treatments produced unpleasant side effects, CBD oil can be an effective solution. It will help the skin moderate its oil production, reduce inflammation on the skin, and will not cause any significant side effects to the user.

CBD oil skin-care products are in the form of oils, creams, and scrubs. There are no directions for use, which allows all-day use. None of the products have THC, even in traces.

Chapter 13: CBD Oil's Neuroprotective Characteristics

Besides all the benefits of CBD oil discussed, it is amazing to learn that the oil also has neuroprotective properties. Having neuroprotective properties means that CBD shelters the brain by promoting cellular repair and healthy brain operations. The United States National Institute of Health acknowledges this therapeutic benefit too.

CBD oil's neuroprotective characteristics obligate it to work towards preventing damage to the central nervous system and to the brain. It encourages the production and development of new neuron cells. It is possible for oxidative stress from genetic disorders, autoimmune conditions, ischemia, and traumatic blows to the head to cause momentary or even perpetual neural damage. However, CBD is able to prevent this from happening and to quicken recovery. From this information, it would seem that CBD would be of great benefit if used therapeutically to treat spinal cord diseases, brain injuries, spinal cord injuries, and strokes.

CBD oil would also prove useful in preventing and controlling the advancement of various neurological disorders like epilepsy, amyotrophic lateral sclerosis, Parkinson's disease, and multiple sclerosis. Although the existing evidence does not fully address effectively how CBD would ensure both neuron and cell health, there is evidence to show that CBD significantly minimizes damage to cells and neurons, thereby encouraging healing.

A number of medical studies have looked into the use of CBD to treat traumatic brain injuries and Chronic Traumatic Encephalopathy. These kinds of injuries to the brain are common in sports. In reality, the sports and recreation industries in the United States report 1.6 million to 3.8 million cases of concussions every year. These injuries are often treated through rehabilitation, self-care, and a prescription of pain medication. However, rather than numbing the pain with prescription pills, perhaps doctors should look into taking up CBD because of its proven neuroprotective properties.

The effectiveness of CBD in treating concussions has been proven. Results drawn from a bunch of medical studies conducted in the past 20 years provide enough evidence. Each of these studies examined the efficacy of CBD in treating persons who suffered various kinds of traumatic brain injuries.

One of these studies is the very same that the government of the United States to validate its claim that CBD is neuroprotective. The study was conducted in 1998 and the results concluded that CBD prevented the death of cells for rats prompted with glutamate neurotoxicity. The study concluded that CBD and other cannabinoids like THC are powerful antioxidants that protect neurons in the brain because they were able to prevent a glutamate-induced death without having to activate cannabinoid receptors.
A second study conducted in 2012 reached a conclusion and the researchers reported that after they had administered CBD following hypoxia-ischemia injury to newborn rats, the CBD provided long-term neuroprotection which allowed their brains to remain functional to a larger extent than they could have if they were allowed to recover histologically. The scientists observed that although CBD causes the healing effects, it did not leave behind any side effects. The results of this study emphasized the usefulness of CBD as a neuroprotector for neonatal hypoxia-ischemia.

A study conducted in 2014 found that CBD went ahead to resolve cognitive impairment that had been induced artificially in mice. The study confirmed CBD's protective effect on the death of neurons that was induced by ischemia. By extension, this shows that CBD would equally be effective in providing therapeutic effects to persons suffering from brain ischemia.

In 2017, a study conducted brought forth results indicating that CBD brings down brain damage and guides it into functional recovery. The study reached this conclusion after observing that administering CBD after brain injury had reduced the loss of neurons, modulated apoptosis, toxicity, and inflammation in the brain leading to functional recovery.

A 2018 review of literature discussing the neurological benefits of cannabinoids concluded that going by the results of animal studies after administering CBD following a head injury, CBD effectively reduced the possibility of having short-term brain damage. It improved metabolic activity in the brain, decreased seizures and brain edema, and reduced the extent of cerebral hemodynamic impairment. The researcher thought the benefits originated from CBD's ability to raise anandamide levels in the brain.

The studies above are proof that CBD has neuroprotective properties that would be beneficial in the treatment of head injuries and other neurodegenerating conditions.

Recommended CBD Schedule for Treating Brain Injuries

When determining the CBD dosage for an illness or a disease like a traumatic brain injury, it is important that CBD is used regularly to provide maximum relief. This means that it should be used for its preventative properties first before it is taken up to manage acute symptoms when they come up. Prevention is more important than symptom management. Patients taking CBD should include it in their daily intake, as they would a dietary supplement, to allow the body to maintain a baseline CBD concentration.

To experience success in the management of brain injury symptoms, patients should ingest full spectrum CBD oil every day, preferably in the form of gel capsules or tinctures. CBD is present in both of these product forms but the difference is only in the dosage and the application. One is taken in the form of pills, while the other in the form of sublingual tinctures.

Persons with brain injuries are advised to begin taking CBD oil starting with a 15mg CBD dosage per day and if this amount does not bring relief, they can increase the dosage by 5-10 mg until they reach optimal dosage when the effects can be felt. Gel capsules, as you will note, are prefilled with either 15mg or 25 mg CBD per capsule. There is no harm if you take 25mg per day above the recommended 15mg. A CBD overdose does not have any serious effects. After ingesting CBD oil, patients should expect to feel some relief setting in and this should last a few hours. Some people even feel the relief all day. However, it is important to note that CBD does not cause relief immediately, it may even take 90 minutes sometimes.

In case the brain injury or illness symptoms are flaring up, many people feel the need to take something to manage them, in addition to their daily dosage. Regardless of what has triggered the symptoms, flare-ups are best managed using vaporized CBD. Vape CBD offers relief almost immediately due to the method of ingesting and the fact that the vape is a pure CBD isolate. However, patients that do not have or do not like vaporizers can still take pills or use tinctures, only being careful to note that those could take some time to offer relief, unlike vaporizing.

From the discussions and the review of studies above, it is clear that CBD would make a useful shield that would protect the brain from neurodegeneration after an injury or infection by disease.

Chapter 14: Other CBD Oil Benefits

CBD oil has so many advantages and the previous chapters have barely scratched the surface. This chapter briefly talks about other benefits that CBD oil consumers can derive from the product besides those already discussed.

They include:

CBD oil helps persons trying to stop smoking
There has been a talk going around that people trying to quit smoking could find CBD oil useful in their endeavor. A small study published in the Addictive Behaviors journal in 2013 confirmed the legitimacy of this claim.

In the study, a sample of 24 smokers received inhalers, some with a placebo substance and others with CBD. The smokers were encouraged to inhale the content for a week throughout the day, whenever the urge to smoke resurfaced. Those inhaling the placebo substance did not notice a reduction in the number of cigarettes they smoked during the week, but those who used the CBD inhaler notices a reduction by about 40%.

The results from this study suggest that CBD has the potential to be used in the treatment of nicotine addiction. However, the results are only preliminary. However, the results are receiving backing from scientists and medical experts. For example, a John Hopkins University professor and cannabis researcher moved his weight behind the study findings but agreed that there needs to be conducted larger long-term studies to confirm that CBD would have long-lasting positive effects on smokers looking to quit the habit.

CBD oil treats Autism
Parents whose children are autistic are now looking towards CBD oil as a potential treatment option for their children, although not much research has been done to confirm this claim.

The speculations behind CBD oil's potential to treat autism are coming from the cannabinoid's ability to interact with the endocannabinoid system in the body, which can be of benefit to autistic persons. The endocannabinoid system plays a role in modeling a person's social behavior, reward processing, and day-to-day rhythm. A research is underway to confirm the effect that CBD could have on autism therapy. Positive results will bring relief and anticipation to parents, their children, and to researchers as well.

However, besides the fact that there have been no human subjects in the studies examining the suitability of CBD for autism, another matter should concern both parents and the patients and prompt them to reconsider their options. The CBD industry is wildly unregulated, especially due to differences in laws between states. In addition, even if manufacturers indicate the ingredients of their oils on the labels, there is not a definite way to confirm that this is true. Patients have to go with customer reviews and the manufacturer's' market size to determine if the product is effective or not. This trial-and-error game should not be used on autistic patients, especially now that research studying CBD and autism is yet to materialize.

A study of some of the CBD oils in the market today found that some CBD products have significant THC levels that could cause unpleasant effects such as getting a child high.

In general, the laws surrounding the use of CBD oil are not yet streamlined and anyone thinking of taking CBD oil should do so with caution, autistic or not.

CBD oil in making skin-care products

We already discussed the use of CBD oil to treat acne, but acne treatment is not the only skin and beauty-related use for CBD oil. CBD's anti-inflammatory characteristics are the reasons why the beauty industry is now looking towards CBD oil as a new active ingredient in anti-aging treatments in the spa and in skincare products.

A New York-based dermatologist recently confirmed that CBD oil has a rich fatty acid deposit among other nutrients that would benefit the skin. The oil also improves skin hydration and reduces the loss of moisture to prevent drying out and flaky skin.

CBD oil can be a treatment for Seizure Disorders
Although there is yet to be enough supporting evidence, CBD oil is said to be helpful to children who experience rare seizure disorders. Epidiolex, a drug derived from CBD, is currently undergoing clinical trials to determine whether it would be effective in reducing seizures for children with either of the two rate kinds of epilepsy – Dravet syndrome and Lennox-Gastaut syndrome. In fact, the FDA has given a go-ahead, allowing the drug to be prescribed to patients suffering from the two forms of epilepsy once the trials are completed.

Using CBD oil shields and heals the skin
The highest number of CB2 receptors in the body is on the skin. Therefore, when CBD oil is applied topically, whether as a lotion, salve, or oil, the antioxidant component of the CBD oil produces many benefits, among them the repair of skin damaged by environmental toxins and free radicals from UV rays.

CBD-based products to be applied on the skin are also being developed to promote quicker healing of damaged skin. In fact, historical documentation of cannabis usage shows that cannabis extracts were applied to wounds to haste healing for both people and animals in many cultures across the globe.

The use of CBD oils to treat skin cancer is also quickly becoming popular. There are even documented cases of persons whose carcinoma and melanoma was cured through the application of both THC and CBD products. The most popular of these cases is that of Rick Simpson who treated his basal cell carcinoma with CBD oil and has now created a variety of products to help others do the same.

However, before you make the first decision concerning the use of CBD oil, ensure that you seek advice from a CBD oil expert and from a medical doctor on the suitability of CBD oil for your situation.

Using CBD oil protects the bones against breaking and diseases

CBDs expedite the process of bone metabolism, which ensures that bones remain healthy and strong as time passes. The bone metabolism process is the process through which bone material is replaced with new material, a small proportion per year. In particular, CBD blocks the enzymes that attempt to destroy the compounds that build the bones. This reduces the risk of developing bone diseases that come with age such as osteoarthritis and osteoporosis. In both of these cases, the body no longer has the ability to create cartilage and bone cells, but the CBD helps to speed up the process of formation of new cells, which is how it has come to be known as a healer of bones.

The new bones get a stronger callus than normal, decreasing the likelihood that the bone could fracture again. Bones of patients who take CBD oils are 35% to 50% stronger than the bones of people who do not take any form of treatment.

Using CBD oil reduces the intensity of childhood epilepsy

Although this quality is discussed slightly in a previous chapter, drug-resistant children who experience neurological disorders like epilepsy that causes them to have seizures can take CBD oil. CBD has anti-seizure characteristics and the body does not become tolerant of it.

In a study that the New England Journal of Medicine published, CBD was seen to reduce seizure frequencies 23 % better than a placebo.

It is exciting to see a natural remedy beating pharmaceutical products in providing fast relief. The FDA is also now recognizing the unique qualities of CBD oils and CBD-based products. For example, FDA cleared the first ever drug extracted from the cannabis plant. There now seems to be a ray of hope that the FDA will be clearing CBD oil and declaring its use in the treatment of diseases legal.

In 2014, researchers from Stanford University approached a group of patents through their Facebook group, a group made up of parents who share experiences they have had on the use of CBD to treat their children's seizures. Nineteen of these cases met the inclusion criteria, which was based on two distinct factors – a clear clinical diagnosis of epilepsy and an ongoing use of CBD-enriched cannabis.

On average, the parents had each tried 12 different kinds of anti-epileptic drugs before turning to CBD from the cannabis. 16 out of the 19 reported a significant reduction in the number of seizures their child experienced after introducing CBD. Of the sixteen, 2 reported complete freedom from seizure, 8 said the seizures had lowered by more than 80%, while 6 reported a fair 25 to 60 percent reduction.

Other benefits the parents reported their children derived from CBD to include a better mood, increased alertness, and improved sleep. Fatigue and drowsiness were commonly reported as side effects.

Later on, in the same year, the researchers gave preliminary results of a study they did with children who had epilepsies that resisted treatment. The patients had received 98% pure hemp-based CBD oil called Epidiolex, manufactured by GW Pharmaceuticals. After only three months of use, the results came in and 39% of the patients were now enjoying a 50% reduction in seizure frequency, while 32% of the study subjects reported a median reduction.

These preliminary results supported those provided by the Facebook parents and those derived from animal studies, which say that CBD might just be the ideal treatment for epilepsy types that have resisted treatment. It also helps that CBD is well tolerated in the body.

CBD oil lowers oxidative stress in the body
CBD oil helps to address oxidative stress in the human body. Oxidative stress refers to the presence of too many free radicals in the body that the body cannot sufficiently neutralize using antioxidants. Oxidative stress is the precursor of many diseases today. It has become more of a problem today than in the past because the environment is increasingly becoming toxic. CBD oil when consumed steps in and acts as an antioxidant and a neuroprotector. It oxidases the free radicals and protects the brain from neurological damage by the free radicals.

CBD oil helps with Schizophrenia
Schizophrenia is a severe and complicated illness that is best managed using pharmaceutical drugs and therapy. The drugs cause a load of side effects that make the situation even more agonizing. However, people have started taking CBD oils to reduce the intensity of the side effect and a number have reported reduced hallucinations. Research is also now showing that CBD is safe and well-tolerated, which makes it an effective and ideal treatment for psychosis. However, the research has not been adequate for CBD to be used on a clinical basis.

It is important to note that while CBD oil helps reduce psychosis, its psychoactive counterpart THC aggravates psychosis for at-risk patients. Therefore, patients using CBD should ensure that they get the pure oil to avoid a counteractive effect.

CBD oil keeps the gut healthy
CBD oil aids in the repair of leaky or tight junctions of the gut that cause decreased spasmodic activity and reduces the permeability of the intestines, a situation common among persons suffering from irritable bowel syndrome.

CBD oil gets rid of nausea
For a long time, cannabis has been used to suppress nausea and vomiting. Research shows that cannabis caused this effect because it contains two cannabinoids that produced this effect

– THC and CBD. The British Journal of Pharmacology published a study in 2012 in support of this finding saying that CBD oil produced antiemetic and anti-nausea effects when it was fed to rats. Further research has also proven that CBD is diphasic, which means that when taken in low doses, it suppresses the urge to vomit, while in high doses, it increases nausea or simply produces no effect.

CBD oil fights a number of drug-resistant bacteria
Scientists have discovered that cannabinoids like CBD have an unusual intolerance towards bacteria, especially the drug-resistant kinds. This discovery requires further research to determine why and how this works.

A study conducted on rats in 2011 also found that CBD slowed down the progression of tuberculosis. The researchers concluded that this is possible because CBD inhibits T-cell proliferation and not because it has antibacterial properties.

However, whichever mechanism CBD oil uses to destroy bacteria, it is proving to be a potent weapon against resistant strains that have become a consistent problem in the world today.

CBD oil helps to manage Cerebral Palsy Symptoms
An infant develops cerebral palsy when its brain is damaged resulting in serious conditions for the rest of the child's life. Persons with cerebral palsy have a more difficult life than that of ordinary people because it affects coordination and movement, which are some of the most critical functions in a person. There is yet to be a cure for cerebral palsy but researchers are continuously coming up with ways to improve the lives of people living with cerebral palsy.

Cerebral palsy presents itself in a number of symptoms, much of which CBD oil has been known to have the ability to suppress. Therefore, if the oil can suppress the majority of the major ones, the patients can live a more full life.

Some of the developmental issues associated with cerebral

palsy include seizures and fits, sight problems, communication and speech difficulties, learning disabilities, and bladder control problems.

Conventional treatments for cerebral palsy so far have aimed at increasing the patients' independence as much as possible and helping them to live a normal life. Physiotherapy is one of the primary treatments. It is meant to strengthen the patients' muscles so that they are able to move around and do other things that require physical strength.

Speech therapy is meant for patients who experience difficulties in speech, swallowing, and communicating. It is used to better their speech or help them learn alternative ways to communicate. Swallowing techniques are important for patients with feeding issues.

Some patients have had to undergo surgery. Surgery is used to fix issues like restoration of movement that is limited by a tight muscle, to ease walking, to enhance the patient's ability to control the bladder, and to correct the curvature of the spine to improve the patient's posture.

Occupational therapy resolves the problems that patients experience when conducting everyday tasks. It helps to boost self-esteem and independence. Pharmaceutical medication is also issued to combat issues like seizures, muscle stiffness, drooling, and others.

Taking CBD oil resolves many of the issues mentioned. This is because it works on the endocannabinoid system (ECS) which is known to regulate many of the body's physiological functions like regulation of the immune system, inflammation, and pain sensitivity. Some of the cerebral palsy symptoms that CBD helps to resolve to include:

Pain: Cerebral palsy patients occasionally complain of chronic pain in the joints and muscles. However, CBD has analgesic properties and helps to relieve the pain.

Muscle spasms: CBD oil significantly reduces muscle spasms and indeed, Sativex, which is a synthetic cannabis form, is prescribed for persons with multiple sclerosis. People with cerebral palsy often experience muscle spasms and CBD oil could greatly benefit them.

Seizures: seizures are common to persons living with cerebral palsy, affecting 35 to 50 percent of the population. CBD oil is effective in reducing seizures as discussed in the previous chapter.

A few studies have been conducted to confirm the claim that CBD oil has positive implications for cerebral palsy patients. The Wolfson Medical Center carried out once such study to determine the effectiveness of cannabis oils for children with the condition. The results were tremendously positive because CBD oil reduced the intensity of the symptoms and improved the children's overall mood, sleep quality, motor skills, and bowel movements.

In conclusion, cerebral palsy is a tough condition because its effects last a lifetime. It makes a person dependent on round-the-clock care for basic functions like walking and going to the toilet. However, CBD oil treatment as a therapy option could ease the patients' lives by reducing the severity of their symptoms. CBD oil is also very simple to use and can be so even for children. They only need a morning dose and the relief benefits will flow throughout the day.

Patients are cautioned that CBD oil should not replace other forms of treatment but that it should be used simultaneously with them.

CBD oil for Crohn's Disease

Crohn's disease is an inflammatory bowel disease (IBD) that causes inflammation in the digestive tract so that a person experiences extremely painful abdominal pains and diarrhea. The pain and dehydration it brings leave a person feeling weak and fatigued all the time. The disease is also associated with rapid weight loss and malnutrition. Crohn's disease easily leads to life-threatening situations.

Studies conducted have shown that CBD oil is useful for treating many diseases and conditions including those affecting the gut. Once a patient ingests CBD oil, it interacts with receptors in the stomach, the intestines, and the brain. These receptors include CB1, CB2, and serotonin. The receptors, in turn, stimulate the body to prevent conditions like vomiting, nausea, and stomach acid irregularities. This increase reduces irritation in the gut and improves the patient's appetite.

CBD oil is a useful treatment for IBDs because it is a natural compound, has different yet easy ingestion methods, and that it works as effectively as therapy does, or in an even better way.

Chapter 15: Testimonial Stories

Following a review of all possible uses and the expected benefits of using CBD oil, it is only right for you to hear directly from the users themselves. This chapter presents a number of testimonies of persons who used CBD oil and an accurate account of how they felt afterward.

Joseph from Denver

34-year old Joseph Jonas who works as a video producer in Denver says that he has long battled muscle and joint pain he believes he got during his earlier days in sports. Tired of pharmaceutical medications and in fear of developing a dependency, he began looking into natural alternatives. He started experimenting with homemade rubs made of compounds like turmeric and arnica. However, he eventually came across CBD-based rubs.

After hiking, he would apply the rub on his lower back and on his ankles and sit there as if to listen to it penetrating his skin. He also used it once when he sprained his shoulder. The CBD rub effectively brought down the pain and the inflammation in the affected area. Joseph says that every time he has used topical CBD, which has been for many years, he has always had positive results.

Joseph recently started taking CBD oil orally in what he describes simply as an 'amazing' experience. He says that it causes him to feel relaxed in a way that takes away all feelings of anxiety. He says that his body feels mellow and limber in a relaxing kind of way.

When asked to give a more detailed explanation of the feeling he gets when he takes CBD oil orally, he gives a simple "I just feel good" reply but insists that he is not high at all.

Joseph's experience with CBD is common among users. Those who have used it before only have praises for the oil.

Richard Holt, UK

Richard Holt posted his story on UK Telegraph explaining how he got injuries on his legs and how CBD oil has helped bring down the pain considerably.

Richard starts by explaining that his woes started in college when he slept on a top bunk next to an open window. At some point in the night, he tried to get up and instead, began his descent 24 feet down, landing on the concrete below, feet first. He was lucky to survive the fall but his feet were not too lucky. His left heel crushed while the tibia and fibula bones on his right leg detached and shattered. The following weeks saw him go through operations and use plates and screws, in a process that brought unimaginable pain. Although the excruciating pain did not return once the legs were healed, some still high-level pain came from time to time.

Having read about CBD oil, Richard began ingesting it using the sublingual method. The experience he got did not compare with that which he had had with Oxycontin, a common opioid painkiller. The opioid had helped him get through the toughest times because besides relieving the pain, it gave him a fuzzy feeling that made him believe that everything was all right. However, after a while, he would be feeling crushed and groggy again. When he observed this, he decided to stop. Richard describes the process of withdrawal as horrendous. He lived in unspeakable misery for days, so bad that it outweighed the pain he had felt when he first became injured. However, he knew that he had to get off the heavy-duty meds.

Richard forged ahead with his daily CBD dose intake and was soon out of his wheelchair, on to crutches and eventually on his legs. He also got a wife and two children in the process. Three years ago, he started taking martial arts again, a hobby he had abandoned. While the CBD may not have gotten him his new family, Richard acknowledges that it made the difference for him, between sitting down and being able to go for training. The pain in his joints has gone down significantly.

Stephanie LaRue
LaRue's story is considered controversial but worthy to mention among CBD oil success stories. LaRue was diagnosed with breast cancer at 30 years of age. She began chemotherapy sessions but also went about looking or alternative cures. In the process, she discovered the Rick Simpson CBD oil. She used it for some time and her cancer went into remission. For nine years now, Stephanie has been wearing her badge of honor, having beaten cancer.

This story is controversial because there is no scientific proof that the cannabis or hemp-based Rick Simpson oil can cure cancer for humans, although it has done that for mice. However, Stephanie is convinced that this is what saved her life.

Charlotte Figi
Among the stories worthy of honorable mention is that of the young girl Charlotte Figi. Hers was one of the most renowned demonstrations of the effectiveness of cannabis, in an effort to improve the quality of life.

Although her story was discussed in the chapters above, it is worth a repeat. Charlotte had been diagnosed with the Dravet syndrome, a form of epilepsy that causes her to experience more than 300 grand mal seizures every week. These seizures made her body frail and interfered with her growth. The disease made her catatonic and delayed her progress, from speech to walking to other kinds of general development.

Doctors prescribed many forms of standard medication but these could not stand her severe symptoms. Her parents had sought all kinds of help and treatments before they eventually turned their attention to CBD oil.

When they made their daughter ingest the oil, the frequency of the seizures started to drop, almost immediately. With time, Charlotte began to lead a normal life and was able to enjoy all the activities of a five-year-old girl.

In honor of her long struggle with epilepsy before finding the cure in cannabis, the strain of the cannabis from which her cure was extracted was named after her. It is called Charlotte's Web. This strain is often used to treat children with Dravet Syndrome and other forms of epilepsy.

Lynn Cameron, Scotland

In 2013, doctors informed Lynn Cameron that she would only be alive for the next 6 to 18 months. This remark came following an incurable brain tumor diagnosis. After several sessions of radiotherapy and chemotherapy, the 48-year old resilient lady decided to try CBD oil as a last resort to save her life. Incredibly, four years after the official diagnosis, Cameron is still alive. She is now an avid supporter of reforms meant to legalize medicinal use of CBD oil.

Kelsey Clark (My Domaine)

In her blog called My Domaine, Kelsey Clark talks about how CBD oil helped her overcome the anxiety that would cause her to become paranoid. Throughout college, she has had episodes of heightened anxiety that would take away her peace, being a person who can overthink sometimes.

When Kelsey heard about the benefits of CBD oil, particularly of the Charlotte's Web Everyday Plus Hemp Oil, she went digging through the internet for more information. She found out that while CBD does not have a psychoactive effect, it relieves anxiety and makes a person less likely to freak out. She also learned that CBD uses the nervous system to work on the responses associated with increased respiration and heartbeat. In other words, CBD was ideal for making people get out of their heads.

Having done adequate research, Kelsey decided to try CBD oil herself. She squeezed a full dropper under her tongue and waited. In about thirty minutes, she was surprised by how subtle the effect felt. She had expected a hazy feeling but the oil simply made her body relax. Her mind stopped racing, her heart stopped pounding, and her legs stopped kicking restlessly. Eventually, the physical relaxation caused her mind to relax and she drifted to a sound sleep.

As Kelsey continued to take the CBD oil over the next six days, she took note of certain changes. She did not have trouble sleeping in the night, she was more focused and productive at work, and she was less anxious. The results from this first week intrigued her enough that she resolved to continue taking the oil and possibly even raise her dosage a bit.

Landon Riddle, Leukemia
At the age of 2, a young boy, Landon Riddle received a Leukemia diagnosis. The doctors observed that his' was the aggressive type of cancer and they only gave him an 8% chance of survival.

His doctor, Dr. Sanjay Gupta, gave a history of Landon's illness in a video released in August 2013. The doctor said that chemotherapy only made the boy violently ill. Riddle was in constant extreme pain and some nerves in his legs had been damaged too. At some point, he stayed 25 days unable to eat or swallow anything.

Landon's mother decided to try CBD-high cannabis oil she acquired from Realm of Caring as her final stroke meant to save his life. Within the first few weeks of CBD oil treatment, the boy's health shifted dramatically and cancer quickly went into remission.

Due to the sudden change, the effectiveness of the oil and the damage chemotherapy had done, the doctors resolved to let Landon use CBD oil only to keep the Leukemia in remission. Landon Riddle is now a grown boy and is doing remarkably well.

Sophie Ryan, Optic Pathway Glioma
Before the girl even turned two, Sophie Ryan had already received an optic pathway glioma diagnosis. Her doctors were certain that the tumor would not respond well to chemotherapy and they shifted their focus towards ensuring that the tumor would not grow any further.

They turned towards cannabinoids and used a combination of oils with a high concentration of CBD and THC-rich oils. These oils, along with occasional chemotherapy, produced outstanding results. The cysts shrank in size by about 75 to 85 percent and the tumor itself is almost entirely gone. Despite the doctors' confident prediction that the treatment would leave Sophie's left eye blind, the girl maintains full vision. Her mother Tracy is now working to help other patients raise money for similar treatments and there is a constant mushrooming of successes particularly among pediatric patients.

Stan Rutner, Brain and Lung Cancer
Stan Rutner successfully fought non-Hodgkin's lymphoma in the 1980s through conventional treatment methods. Unfortunately, cancer returned more aggressively and attacked his brain and his lungs in 2011. This time around, radiation and chemotherapy were no good and Stan was put on hospice care.

Desperate for some relief, Stan began to ingest cannabis-infused coconut oil to relieve his pain. The change that occurred was dramatic. On seeing this, Stan began taking larger doses of concentrated CBD oil and THC. Beginning in 2013, Stan was declared completely cancer free.

Dennis Hill, Prostate Cancer
Dennis Hill previously worked as a biochemist and specialized in cancer research. However, in 2010, the scientist was diagnosed with an aggressive prostate cancer. Not wanting to put his body through radiation, chemotherapy, or surgery, Dennis began looking into alternative medicine. He learned about the potential benefits of CBD oil and after some bit of research, found that the oil would go well with his body chemistry.

He only took Lupron to slow the rate of tumor growth by reducing testosterone production but the drug could not kill cancer cells directly.

With this treatment alone, Hill had succeeded in beating cancer by early 2011. Cancer returned for a brief moment in 2012, but he relentlessly kicked it out again with cannabinoid therapy.

Michael Cutler, Liver Cancer

Unfortunately, some stories like that of Michael Cutler do not end too well. This man was a popular activist in the UK primarily because of his work with the United Patients Alliance, an organization that seeks to amend the laws and to increase awareness among the people of the medicinal benefits of cannabis.

For the second time, Michael was diagnosed with liver cancer in late 2012. This time, the doctors gave a terminal diagnosis saying that cancer had progressed beyond treatment and that nothing could be done to reverse this. However, Michael was sure that he would overcome cancer and he sought alternative help in CBD oils. After using it for a few months, a biopsy done in May 2014 revealed that Michael was now cancer free.
A few months later, unfortunately, Michael developed lung cancer and this time, he could not procure the CBD oils. He died on the third day of December 2014 according to the United Patients Alliance. His medical journey serves as a demonstration of the brutality and the negative results that occur due to the prohibition of essential treatments and the need for immediate change.

Cash Hyde, Brain Tumor

Another sad case was that of Cash Hyde, the little boy whose case inspired the movement to promote the use of cannabis products on children.

Cash's initial prognosis done in May 2010 revealed that he had Stage IV brain tumor. This diagnosis was very poor and Cash did not show any positive response to chemotherapy. As a last resort, his parents made him ingest CBD oil through his feeding tube and in no time, Cash began experiencing big changes that completely turned his health around. After 8 months, when another test was conducted in January 2011, the doctors declare Cash cancer-free.

Sadly, Cash's family could not secure a constant supply of CBD oil, which was needed as a maintenance dose, and as you would expect, cancer returned. However, this time too, Cash defied the odds and cancer went into remission again. This time too, his maintenance dose ran out, creating room for another cancer attack. This third time, cancer came back and Cash's body could not fight it back.

On the fourteenth day of November 2012, Cash passed away. In his memory, The Cash Hyde Foundation was started to help patients and to create cancer awareness and the healing properties of CBD oil.

Conclusion

Thank you for making it through to the end of *The Ultimate Guide to Hemp CBD Oil: Complete Guide to Dealing with Anxiety, Depression, Diseases, Pain Relief and CBD Legality - Improve Health and Happiness Using this Miraculous Oil.* I hope it was informative and able to provide you with all of the tools you need to achieve your goals whatever they may be.

Certainly, you are amazed by the fact that one product can serve so many purposes yet its use is so restricted. It is must have been sad to see how something so good can face so much opposition and restriction, particularly from those it would benefit.

For many years, many benefits of the cannabis oil have been overlooked, primarily due to its relationship with its THC, its psychoactive counterpart. The cannabis plant has been shunned because, from a social perspective, people who take anything from it begin to 'misbehave'. Others believe that consuming anything that contains THC only worsens a patient's condition instead of correcting it. It is also sad that bureaucracy and legislation have kept people from delving deeper since the benefits of CBD were realized in the 1950s.

However, the current buzz on the benefits of CBD oil is shifting things in the right direction. We are living at a time when people want to be heard, and if more people learn about the CBD oil benefits, they are likely to cause a movement that will see the relaxation of laws that restrict the growth of the cannabis industry and the use of CBD products among the people. It is also likely that the cannabis industry will be more regulated to ensure that the products in the market are legit and offer consumers the benefits promised.

The next step is to start sharing the knowledge you have obtained from this book with others. With enough word around, the people will become more aware of the options available to them. Authorities will begin to ease the limiting laws they have placed on CBD oil manufacturers. Governments will begin to aid research into more CBD oil benefits. In the end, the people shall be more knowledgeable of CBD oil benefits and the oil will be right at their doorsteps.

Finally, if you found this book useful in any way, a review on Amazon is always appreciated!

www.ingramcontent.com/pod-product-compliance
Lightning Source LLC
Chambersburg PA
CBHW072215170526
45158CB00002BA/615

* 9 7 8 1 0 9 1 1 9 6 3 7 7 *